From Harmony to Discord:
A Layman's Guide to Cancer

Nina

Table of Contents

Introduction

<u>1.1.1 An analogy for cancer</u>

Humans are composed of an orchestra of 37.2 trillion microscopic cells working in concert to compose a symphony of life.[1] Symphonies are grand works of art with a variety of instruments simultaneously cooperating to perform a highly regulated and complex sound. Every member reads the same music sheet, but they are only responsible for playing their designated notes. As you can imagine, if one musician is disobedient and plays random notes, the sound from that one member would not be noticeable. But if throughout the course of the song, the proportion of disobedient members grows, it would begin to sound like utter chaos. This analogy can be likened to cancer, where the music sheet is the genome, the notes are genes, and the different instruments are varying cell types in the body. In a Canadian's lifetime, one in two people will experience a phenomenon where a single member of their orchestra will disobey the script, not by choice, but by random chance.[2] Often it begins with a small error that promotes a founder cell to possess one of the hallmarks of cancer, and at this stage it is impossible to detect.[3] That founder cell will divide into daughter cells each holding the same mutation, and their proportion grows as they continue to divide. What is more is they will accumulate further mutations, made worse by genetic instability. The conductor of the orchestra, the immune system, will attempt to restore order by removing rogue members. However, the very same process of random genetic mutation which created and drove these errant cells will also help them adapt to their environmental pressures through natural selection. Eventually the cancer snowballs until the population is large enough to be heard, making the patient's symphony noisy and disarrayed. Oncologists step in to assume the position of conductor, delivering the standard of care in an attempt to reverse entropy. Unfortunately, some instruments are louder than others, and depending on their abundance, current medical practices are insufficient to remove them all. Oncologists desperately need better solutions to silence the madness and return their patient's music back to its original state for everyone to enjoy.

1.1.2 The trouble with cancer

All cancers have distinct characteristics depending on the tissue of origin and in part because of wildly variable mutation profiles, not only between individuals, but even across tumours in the same patient.[4] This is an important reason why existing treatments do not work with everyone, and is also the biggest challenge in developing new medicines. When a malignant tumour is first diagnosed, it is imperative to act quickly. Every day is an opportunity for new mutations to accumulate which advances its genetic complexity, and every day is an opportunity for cancer cells to migrate from the primary site to distal locations across the body. Though largely dependent on the cell type, metastases often form in areas with ramified vasculature such as the lungs, liver, and brain.[5,6] As these metastatic tumours expand, they disrupt the proper functioning of these organs, and most patients die because of metastatic burden. This is why early detection, as well as the stage of progression at diagnosis, have a crucial influence on the patient's prognosis.

1.1.3 Cancer treatment in 2020

Standard of care treatment approaches are individualized based on cancer type and how far it has spread. For decades the three main pillars of cancer therapy have been surgery, radiation therapy, and chemotherapy. Surgery is often necessary, if possible, to remove the primary tumour and accessible metastases. Localized malignant sites can be treated by concentrating high doses of gamma radiation in a region to induce double stranded DNA breaks and apoptosis. However, to treat advanced metastatic disease, systemic chemotherapy is often required to attack cancer cells that have seeded throughout the body. Chemotherapy is notoriously toxic due to its by-stander killing of healthy cells. Furthermore, the host's immune cells also fall victim to the drugs, causing severe immune suppression. Therefore, the specificity and safety of next-generation therapeutics are of utmost importance to reduce sickness and suffering, while maintaining a competent immune response which is an integral component of the patient's fight. Alternative therapies are required due to deficiencies in current treatment approaches which often lead to a poor response, acquired resistance, and relapse.

1.2.1 Emergence of the fourth pillar

Chemotherapy destroys the immune system, but what if instead the focus of cancer treatment is to support it? Doing so might provide a more comprehensive treatment option, and with immune memory there is the potential for cancer vaccination to reduce the odds of relapse. Cancer immunotherapy is a significant area of research in the biomedical scientific community, as it's been well established that the immune system has an integral role in restricting cancer progression and clearing tumours. In a broad sense, the primary function of the immune system is to detect and neutralize foreign biological materials. One of the most important underlying mechanisms occurs during lymphocyte maturation. Developing lymphocytes are produced with a random T-cell or B-cell receptor (TCR or BCR) through V(D)J gene recombination, each with the potential to recognize a distinct peptide epitope.[7] The diversity in this repertoire is estimated to be 1×10^{15} antigen specificities, therefore it is almost certain the developing lymphocyte pool can recognize any and every protein possible.[8] To prevent mature immune cells from reacting to host proteins, maturing lymphocytes undergo a process of positive and negative selection in the thymus to remove those that bind to self-antigens.[9] Theoretically, this means the immune system can attack any protein without an identical amino acid sequence to the host. Foreign biologics with highly dissimilar proteins to humans such as helminths, viruses, and bacteria are particularly vulnerable. Cancer cells are largely tolerated by the immune system because they are derived from host cells. However, as mentioned previously, cancer cells carry a large burden of genetic mutations that ultimately introduce changes in the amino acid sequence of some of its proteins. Its these mutant epitopes, called tumour neoantigens, that can be recognized by the immune system.

<u>1.2.2 Adoptive T-cell transfer</u>

Tumour-associated antigens (TAAs) are at the root of many ongoing experimental cancer immunotherapies. Lymphocyte clonotypes that recognize these TAAs are the key effector cells that attack cancer, especially the $CD8^+$ cytotoxic T-cell populations. A significant amount of these cells concentrate in the tumour to eradicate cancer cells expressing TAAs. One mode of cancer treatment is adoptive T-cell therapy, where T-cells isolated from a resected tumour are then cultured *in vitro* with growth factors to multiply and activate the population. This army of cancer-specific lymphocytes is then reinfused back into the patient in high numbers to respond to other cancer cells remaining in the body. A similar mode of treatment, chimeric antigen receptor (CAR)-T cell therapy, is done the same way except the isolated CD8[+] lymphocytes are genetically engineered with a recombinant TCR that recognizes a preselected TAA. The chimeric antigen receptor rapidly activates the cytotoxic killer functions of the T-cell. In this case, the TAA is not a mutant host protein, but rather a protein that is commonly found to be upregulated in cancer.[10] Both modes of adoptive T-cell therapy have shown promising results in clinical trials and are an active area of research.

<u>1.2.3 Monoclonal antibody therapy</u>

Another rapidly advancing immunotherapy that has effectively translated into the clinic is monoclonal antibody therapy, in particular immune checkpoint blockade. Immunoglobulins, or antibodies, are protein complexes secreted from activated B lymphocytes with identical specificity to the BCR. Antibodies can be chemically conjugated to a cytotoxic drug, and due to the cancer-specificity of the antibody it is an effective means of drug delivery to tumours. Antibodies can also be used to interrupt the interaction of a protein with its ligand. As mentioned, cancer-specific CD8[+] lymphocytes as well as other immune cells are found throughout a tumour, however they are often induced into a resting inactive state. Originally these cells were competent in performing their cytotoxic functions, but began to upregulate programmed cell death protein 1 (PD1) expression as a negative feedback loop. PD1 on the CD8[+] T-cells (and other immune cells) binds with the PD-L1 ligand on cancer cells, and this interaction inhibits signalling in the T-cell. Antibodies targeting PD1 or PD-L1 can disrupt this interaction, thereby "releasing the brakes" on the T-cell and enabling it to carry out its functions for a prolonged period of time.[11] This mode of treatment, called immune checkpoint blockade, has had remarkable success with favourable toxicity profiles in treating advanced recurrent disease and has quickly progressed though clinical trials. Now, antibodies targeting cytotoxic T-lymphocyte-associated protein 4 (CTLA-4), a checkpoint protein similar to PD1, have been approved for first-line treatment in melanoma patients.[12] Scientists involved in the discovery of these proteins and its application in monoclonal antibody therapy were awarded the Nobel Prize in Physiology and Medicine in 2018.[13]

Following the success of checkpoint blockade in the clinic, there has been a recent surge of interest to find appropriate therapies to deliver in combination. Therapies that attract lymphocytes to the tumour are suitable candidates due to its mechanism of action, and viruses are effective at doing so because of their highly immunostimulatory nature. Not every virus would be appropriate in this context, rather ones that can localize to tumours are ideal. Sure enough, oncolytic viruses (OVs) have had success in combination with checkpoint inhibitors.[14–17]

<u>1.2.4 Oncolytic viruses</u>

OVs are replication competent viral vectors that preferentially infect cancer cells. A variety of viruses have this capability through different mechanisms. For example, cancer cells occasionally have defects in the interferon pathway which creates an ideal environment for interferon-sensitive viruses like vesicular stomatitis virus (VSV) to replicate.[18] In the case of VSV, this specificity was further improved through genetic modification of one of its genes, yielding the current OV platform VSVΔ51.[19] Similarly, vaccinia virus' (VacV) cancer-selectivity can be improved through genetic manipulation of one of its genes, thymidine kinase.[20] Tumour tropism can also be redirected by disrupting a viral gene used for entry and replacing it with a targeting ligand.[21]

Since viruses carry and express genetic material, this opens the opportunity to genetically engineer the vectors for localized transgene expression in tumours. Furthermore, OVs directly lyse cancer cells or otherwise kill them by triggering apoptosis. Their oncotropism, combined with their utility as gene delivery vectors, oncolytic capabilities, immunostimulatory nature, and propagation after an initial dose are ideal characteristics for a foundation to develop next-generation anti-cancer therapeutics. The field of oncolytic virotherapy is derived from historical observations that cancer patients with hematologic malignancies occasionally experienced remission that coincided with natural viral infections.[22] There are several case reports of leukemias, Hodgkin's lymphoma, and Burkitt's lymphoma regressing after a bout with measles, suggesting that its causative organism, Measles virus (MeV), has anticancer activity.[23]

1.3.1 Introduction to measles

Measles is a highly contagious infectious disease which transmits through respiratory droplets infecting ten million people annually.[24,25] The basic reproduction number (R_0) is defined as the number of secondary cases of infectious disease that can be traced back to a primary case in a completely susceptible population. In other words, it is a measure of how many people become infected by one sick person, so R_0 is a proxy for contagiousness. The estimated R_0 for MeV ranges between 15-20.[24,26] As a point of comparison, the currently pandemic SARS-CoV-2 has an estimated R_0 between 2.24-3.58.[27] SARS-CoV-2 has spread to almost every country in the world seemingly overnight, and is continuing to surge despite an unprecedented global effort to curb its spread. Also, Influenza virus has an R_0 between 1.4-4.[24] So compared to other viruses circulating in the population, MeV is exceptionally contagious.

Measles patients present with a fever, severe cough, and Koplik spots, followed by a maculopapular rash on the face which spreads cephalocaudally.[24,28] Another important hallmark is transient immune suppression which can lead to opportunistic infections accounting for high mortality.[29] In rare cases, measles can cause a variety of neurological complications during or long after the disease has resolved. One of these conditions, subacute sclerosing panencephalitis (SSPE), is important to highlight as it later relates to this book. SSPE is a slowly progressive neurodegenerative disorder. Tissue damage in the brain occurs due to the inflammatory response to a mutated MeV infecting the patient's neurons.[30] Persistent measles infection in the brain occurs years after acute measles infection, culminating in cognitive decline, gait abnormalities and eventually a vegetative state and death.[29,30]

Susceptible infants and children are at highest risk of developing severe complications and fatal disease, including SSPE.[24,28,30] Pneumonia is the cause of death in 60% of measles-related deaths, which totaled 160,000 in 2018.[25,28] A majority of the ten million cases and 160,000 deaths are in low-income African and Asian countries where gaps in vaccination coverage exist due to resource-constrained health care systems.[30] Measles has been less prevalent in Canada and other high-income developed countries in the postvaccination era. This is because the measles-mumps-rubella (MMR) vaccine is nearly 100% effective at preventing measles when given in two doses at an appropriate interval in children aged one year or older, and 93% of the population must be immunized to preserve herd immunity.[28] This is being threatened by anti-vaccination sentiments and misinformation that have flourished on social media in recent decades.[31] As a result, MMR immunization rates have dropped as low as 60% in some regions of developed countries, and the consequence has been multiple measles outbreaks.[32] In these epidemics, susceptible individuals will become infected and develop lifelong immunity to reinfection, temporarily restoring population immunity.[24]

<u>1.3.2 Live attenuated measles vaccines</u>

Active immunization is achieved through subcutaneous injection of a small dose (10^3 fifty-percent tissue culture infective dose ($TCID_{50}$)) of live attenuated MeV to induce protective levels of anti-measles antibodies.[23,24] Most measles vaccines are laboratory-adapted sub-strains of the Edmonston lineage (MeV-Edm) which was first isolated from a child named David Edmonston in 1954.[33] MeV-Edm lost its pathogenicity after serial passaging in tissue culture but still had side effects in naïve children.[23] Further passaging in chicken embryo fibroblasts gave rise to the more attenuated MeV-Moraten and Edmonston-Zagreb strains which were ultimately used to try to eradicate measles in the United States and Europe respectively.[23] MeV-Edm derivatives have since showcased an excellent safety profile in over one billion vaccinated individuals worldwide, with minimal side effects and no reported cases of reversion to wildtype MeV.[24]

Wild-type MeV enters immune and epithelial cells through two receptors, signalling lymphocyte-activation molecule family member 1 (SLAMF1)/CD150 and PVRL4/nectin-4 respectively.[34,35] Early infection is established in SLAMF1-expressing immune cells (such as macrophages) in the respiratory tract followed by spread to lymphoid tissues that are rich in SLAMF1+ lymphocytes.[29] Infected immune cells transport the virus systemically, likely shedding virus to nearby nectin-4-expressing epithelial cells and keratinocytes. Unique to the laboratory-adapted strains is a third entry receptor that MeV-Edm acquired from an N481Y amino acid substitution in its envelope protein during serial passaging of wild-type virus for vaccine development.[36] This receptor is the membrane cofactor protein (MCP/CD46), which is ubiquitously expressed on all nucleated cells, therefore giving MeV-Edm a much wider tropism than its wild-type counterpart.

<u>1.3.3 MeV genome</u>

Measles virus is the prototypical member of the genus *Morbillivirus* in the family *Paramyxoviridae*. Like all paramyxoviruses, its virions are enveloped and pleomorphic in shape, containing a non-segmented, single-stranded RNA genome of negative polarity.[37] Its genome is typically 15,894 nucleotides in length and encodes six structural proteins (N,P,M,F,H, and L), and two accessory proteins (V and C) generated from RNA editing or the use of an alternative ORF in the P gene to serve as virulence factors *in vivo*.[38,39] The genome length is a multiple of six, and this is because the nucleoprotein (N) coats the RNA strand forming the ribonucleoprotein complexes with six nucleotides bound to each N monomer.[40] The "rule of six" is preferred for optimal paramyxovirus genome replication, as nonpolyhexameric lengths replicate less efficiently and evolve correcting mutations to conform to this rule.[41] *P* gene RNA editing and hexameric genome lengths are linked in paramyxoviruses, because they are required for RNA dependent RNA polymerase (RdRp) initiation at the genome's 3' end.[42] The RdRp complex is composed of the large protein (L) complexed with homo-tetrameric phosphoprotein (P), where the L subunit possesses enzymatic activity for transcription and replication, and P mediates binding to the N-encapsidated viral RNA genome.[43]

1.3.4 MeV syncytiogenesis

The last three MeV genes warrant greater introduction as their cooperation is particularly relevant to this book. Namely these are the matrix (*M*), fusion (*F*), and haemagglutinin (*H*) genes. Firstly, the *F* and *H* (or *G/HN*) genes are glycoproteins anchored in the envelope of all paramyxoviruses and mediate virus-cell and cell-cell fusion. The tetrameric H protein varies considerably across paramyxovirus subtypes and is responsible for recognizing its cognate host-cell receptors for attachment, and therefore the virus' tropism. The trimeric F protein is more conserved across paramyxoviruses and interacts with H, triggering membrane fusion upon conformational changes from H binding to its receptor.[44] This process is essential for viral entry, by inducing virus-cell fusion to release the viral genome into the host cytoplasm. Upon infecting the cell, the glycoproteins are expressed and traffic to the host plasma membrane. F is inert at first and must be endocytosed and cleaved by furin-like peptidases into two disulfide-linked subunits which are then biologically active.[44] Fusion-ready membrane-bound F/H complexes can then mediate cell-cell fusion between the infected cell and neighbouring naïve cells expressing the viral receptor. As this process continues, the result is large multi-nucleated cells called syncytia which is one mechanism of MeV intercellular spread.

1.3.5 MeV egress and budding

Another mechanism of inter-cellular spread is through assembly and budding of infectious particles that diffuse to distal uninfected cells. The key gene in this process is the matrix protein (M) that tethers the ribonucleoprotein complexes to the cytoplasmic tails of the glycoproteins at the inner side of the plasma membrane, thereby joining the virus' cargo to its envelope. This interaction between the matrix protein and glycoproteins is

necessary 11

for assembly, but also downregulates glycoprotein-mediated cell-cell fusion.[45] M binding to the cytoplasmic tails of F and H induces a conformational change that disables their fusion activity while infectious particles are formed.[45,46] A clean demonstration of this is shown by co-transfecting M in fusion assays, where M expression inhibits glycoprotein mediated fusion.[46–48] In fact, a matrix-less MeV is assembly-defective but produces dramatically larger syncytia,[49] likely due to the glycoproteins being completely uninhibited. These features are consistent with MeV isolates taken from SSPE patients, which similarly bud less virus and are more fusogenic due to characteristic hypermutation in the *M* gene or cytoplasmic tails *of F* and *H*.[45,50]

Not much is known about the mechanism of matrix protein trafficking, except that the actin cytoskeleton is important, annexin A2 (*ANXA2*) is involved, and it's ESCRT-independent.[51–53] Modulating cytoskeletal dynamics impairs MeV M trafficking and reduces its accumulation at the plasma membrane, meanwhile glycoprotein trafficking is unaffected, which results in the characteristic hyperfusogenic assembly-defective phenotype.[53] Mutations that affect M protein stability, thereby increasing its turnover, reduces M surface accumulation and also leads to the same phenotype.[50]

1.4.1 Oncolytic virus monotherapy in the clinic

Important studies using MeV-Edm strains as antitumour agents emerged at the turn of the 21st century during a boom of oncolytic virus research. MeV-Edm was first studied in B-cell non-Hodgkin's lymphoma and successfully regressed large established xenografts *in vivo*.[54] In this study, expression of the MeV attachment receptor, CD46, was confirmed in the lymphoma cell lines that were efficiently infected *in vitro*. Serendipitously, it was later found that CD46 is highly expressed on most cancer cells, presumably as an adaptation to inactivate autologous complement-mediated attack.[55] Since CD46 is involved in the attachment and entry of MeV-Edm, this is one of the proposed mechanisms for its natural oncotropism.

To date, many OVs have been translated into early and late phase clinical trials and have demonstrated favourable safety and tolerability, confirming this therapy modality is appropriate for human application. However, these first-generation OVs have had limited success in most patients. PVS-RIPO is a noteworthy OV that has shown strong efficacy. It is a genetically modified poliovirus designed to treat advanced recurrent glioblastoma. In a recent trial, 19% of patients treated with PVS-RIPO had severe adverse side effects grade three or higher, however, 21% of patients survived with durable complete remission until the end of the 72-month study.[56] In comparison, the survival rate with historical controls is only 4% after 72-months, so the results of this study show a ground-breaking improvement over the standard of care. With such promising efficacy, PVS-RIPO received breakthrough status from the United States Food and Drug Administration which will expedite the development and assessment of this therapy.

So far, three different measles virus constructs have been tested in more than 150 cancer patients, and while many patients benefit from a clinical response and stable disease, all but one case had eventually succumbed to their disease.[24] The survivor was a multiple myeloma patient who was refractory to all available treatments, but experienced complete remission after one intravenous infusion of 10^{11} TCID$_{50}$ MeV-NIS.[57] NIS stands for sodium iodine symporter, and it was genetically encoded into the MeV genome as a means of non-invasive imaging using radioiodine to track MeV replication in lesions.[58] Another transgene encoded into a clinical MeV construct is carcinoembryonic antigen (CEA), a soluble marker that enables quantitative monitoring of virus replication *in vivo*.[59] The only other oncolytic MeV tested in humans was an unmodified Edmonston-Zagreb strain.[60] Reporter transgenes serve an important role in understanding the dynamics of MeV infection in human cancers *in* vivo, but improved outcomes will not be seen until therapeutic transgenes are used to augment the virus' anticancer effects. There has been considerable focus in the field to find creative and exciting ideas to meet this end, leading to an abundance of new promising preclinical studies.

<u>1.4.2 Oncolytic virus transgenes</u>

NIS has a supplementary capacity to be used as a therapeutic transgene in radiovirotherapy by driving intracellular uptake of ^{131}I isotopes in infected cells, but this has only been studied preclinically.[61] Synergy between MeV-NIS and ^{131}I radiotherapy has been shown in mice with subcutaneous human xenografts of pancreatic adenocarcinoma, medulloblastoma, prostate cancer, squamous cell cancer of the head and neck, and anaplastic thyroid cancer.[61–65] This approach leverages the capacity of oncolytic viruses to localize NIS expression inside cancer cells. Similarly, tumour-restricted activation of chemotherapeutics has been explored by encoding prodrug convertases into the oncolytic MeV genome. The first virally-encoded prodrug convertases used *Escherichia coli* purine nucleotide phosphorylase in conjunction with systemic fludarabine treatment, which gets processed exclusively inside the tumour to generate toxic ATP analogs.[66–68] Due to toxicity concerns from systemic fludarabine administration, current chemovirotherapeutic strategies utilize the super cytosine deaminase (SCD) transgene instead, which is a fusion protein of the yeast-derived cytosine deaminase and uracil phosphoribosyltransferase.[69–72] Tumour-restricted expression of SCD converts the prodrug 5-fluorocystosine into 5-fluorouracil then 5-fluorouridine monophosphate (5-FUMP), which cellular enzymes then process into toxic metabolites that interfere with DNA repair, as well as DNA, RNA, and protein synthesis.[69]

Recently, there has been substantial preclinical research into immunomodulation with transgenes. Grote *et al.* suspected the host inflammatory response, particularly neutrophils, were important to the anticancer effect seen in early oncolytic MeV studies.[73] To potentiate the functions of neutrophils, cytokine granulocyte-macrophage colony stimulating factor (GM-CSF) was encoded into MeV and tested in a severe combined immunodeficient (SCID) mouse model of human lymphoma. MeV-GM-CSF outperformed unmodified MeV, which correlated with neutrophil infiltration in the tumour. However, SCID mice lack a functional adaptive immune system, which was becoming recognized as an important component of virotherapy. Grossardt *et al.* addressed this in an immunocompetent murine colon adenocarcinoma model using transgenic MC38cea cells permissive to retargeted MeV-antiCEA.[74] MeV-antiCEA armed with GM-CSF not only enhanced median overall survival, but remarkably a third of the mice were effectively cured. These mice rejected tumours upon rechallenge, demonstrating a durable adaptive immune response and cancer-specific immunization.[74] GM-CSF has since translated into the clinic, as it is encoded in the first globally-approved oncolytic virus Talimogene laherparevec.

As mentioned previously, oncolytic viruses are an ideal partner for combination therapy with immune checkpoint inhibitors. Engeland and colleagues virally-encoded PDL-1 and CTLA-4 antibodies into MeV to create a functional monotherapy that demonstrated synergy in an immunocompetent B16 mouse model.[15] Bi-specific T-cell engagers (BiTes) also have the capacity to engage TILs with cancer cells. BiTes are covalently linked single-chain variable fragments with dual specificity for T-cells and a preselected tumour antigen, thereby bringing them in proximity to activate the T-cell.[75] MeV expressing BiTes induced significant infiltration of CD8[+] cytotoxic T-cells in a B16-CD20-CD46 mouse model.[76] In another study by the same group, MeV-IL-12 likewise enhanced the abundance of CD8[+] TILs, and depletion experiments showed this T-cell subtype was crucial for its efficacy.[77]

<u>1.4.3 RNA interference</u>

To date, most therapeutic transgenes have been protein-coding, essentially introducing or overexpressing a beneficial protein in a system. However, transgenes which interfere with a target protein that is already present in the system is lacking. Such a technology would enable local disruption of signalling pathways in the tumour. RNA interference (RNAi) is a particularly powerful and versatile tool to downregulate a gene by carefully designing target-specific complementary oligonucleotides. In the laboratory, RNA interference is common to study the outcome from transiently suppressing a target gene using small interfering RNAs (siRNAs) or stably expressing short hairpin RNAs (shRNAs) from virally transduced cells. These technologies mimic endogenous micoRNAs naturally present within cells and use the same method of silencing. The final structure of the microRNA is a double-stranded RNA duplex ~22 nucleotides in length with one strand (the guide) used as a template in the RNA-induced silencing complex (RISC) for miRNA-target recognition. Specificity relies on sequence complementarity between the guide strand and target mRNA transcript, where nucleotides 2-7 of the miRNA guide strand are critically important.[78] A perfect match is required in this region (called the "seed" region), whereas pairing outside of the seed has a degree of flexibility to allow for some mismatches. Sequence features outside of the seed region influence the degree of knockdown efficiency, such as GC composition.[78–80] After the mature microRNA is loaded into RISC, the complex searches for target mRNAs which are then cleaved upon successful RISC:target association.[80] After mRNA cleavage, the product is released from the complex and subsequently degraded, thereby decreasing target mRNA and protein levels. Alternatively, if mRNA cleavage does not occur, RISC complex association to the mRNA can stall ribosome translation, thereby decreasing protein levels through translational repression without effecting mRNA abundance.[81]

Gene-silencing mediated by endogenous microRNAs has been used to control the tropism of viral gene-delivery vectors. The target site of tissue-specific microRNAs is encoded into the genome of lentiviral or oncolytic viral vectors to improve safety by reducing infection of unintended cells.[82,83] For example, with OVs, microRNAs that are highly expressed in healthy tissues but poorly expressed in cancer are selected. What is yet to be accomplished is encoding functional microRNAs into oncolytic MeV as a therapeutic transgene. A limitation for cytoplasmic viral vectors, such as MeV, is that microRNA processing begins in the nucleus. Furthermore, endogenous microRNAs often target multiple mRNAs.[84] To both tailor and refine their specificity, artificial microRNAs (amiRNAs) can be produced by replacing the biologically active sequence of a mature microRNA within the hairpin of an endogenous primary microRNA transcript.[85,86] The new stem sequence is designed with perfect complementarity to a target gene, therefore amiRNAs are a flexible platform for post-transcriptional gene regulation. Multiple hairpins can also be engineered into microRNA clusters to suppress multiple targets.[86]

Theoretically, target knockdown should be highly specific, but in practice, RNAi often unintentionally suppresses off-target mRNAs through seed region complementarity.[87] There are also many examples of off-target microRNA suppression using non-canonical target sites.[88]

<u>1.4.4 Targeting RIG-I and the interferon pathway</u>

The aim of encoding amiRNAs into oncolytic MeV is to arm the virus with a therapeutic transgene which can be modified to suppress a specific gene in cancer. amiRNA expression and target knockdown would be tumour-restricted due to the inherent oncotropism of oncolytic MeV. We focused on targeting antiviral restriction factors to give the virus a replicative advantage in cancer. An important antiviral pathway that interferes with MeV replication is the interferon response.[89,90] The interferon pathway is an innate antiviral immune response that is triggered upon recognition of pathogen associated molecular patterns (PAMPs). The PAMPs of MeV are 5' triphosphate-containing double-stranded RNAs which are recognized by the host pattern recognition receptor (PRR) retinoic acid inducible gene I (RIG-I).[91] Other important PRRs are melanoma differentiation associated protein 5 (MDA5) and laboratory of genetics and physiology 2 (LGP2).[91] Upon RIG-I binding to a PAMP, the C-terminal domain (CTD) unfolds and reveals the caspase activation and recruitment domains (CARDs) at its N-terminus.[92,93] The CARD domains (exons 1-5 of RIG-I) contain multiple lysine residues which are then exposed after release of the CTD to become poly-K63-ubiquitinated. The polyubiquitinated CARD domains then associate to mitochondrial antiviral signalling protein (MAVS).[94] The downstream signalling cascade ends in the activation of transcription factors which drive interferon stimulated gene (ISG) expression. ISGs function to inhibit viral replication and induce neighbouring cells into an antiviral state. Interfering with this pathway should help boost MeV replication in cancer cells, which would ultimately improve MeV oncolysis and may also benefit other aspects of the therapy such as the anti-cancer immune response. The hypothesis was that <u>the innate immune response could be silenced by engineering the MeV genome to express amiRNAs targeting RIG-I, thereby improving oncolytic MeV replication in cancer cells compared to unmodified vectors.</u> The versatility of redirecting the target sequence in the amiRNA cassette towards other host factors would open the opportunity generate novel MeV vectors in the future which can target selected genes inside tumours.

Materials and Methods

<u>1. Cell lines and virus</u>

GM-38 fibroblasts were received from Dr. Carolina Ilkow (Ottawa Hospital Research Institute, Ottawa, Canada) and were maintained in Dulbecco's Modified Eagle Medium (DMEM) (Corning, NY, USA) supplemented with 2% fetal bovine serum. All other cell lines were received courtesy of Dr. John Bell (Ottawa Hospital Research Institute, Ottawa, Canada) and were maintained in DMEM + 10% FBS. Cell lines were verified to be free from mycoplasma contamination with the PCR Mycoplasma Detection Kit (abmGood, BC, Canada) prior to expansion and storage at -120°C. A549 RIG$^{-/-}$ CRISPR KO cells were received from Dr. Marco Binder (National Center for Tumour Diseases Heidelberg, Heidelberg, Germany). MeV ld-EGFP was rescued from a plasmid containing the genome of Schwarz strain MeV harbouring the EGFP marker in an additional transcription unit upstream of the *N* gene. MeV P-Fluc was rescued from a plasmid containing the genome of Schwarz strain MeV harbouring the firefly luciferase luminescent marker in an additional transcription unit upstream of the *P* gene. Aliquots of VacV-GFP, HSV-1-GFP, and VSV-GFP were gifted from Dr. Tommy Alain (Children's Hospital of Eastern Ontario Research Institute, Ottawa, Canada) to perform the live cell imaging experiments. The HSV-1-GFP virus is an ΔICP0 (infected cell protein 0) mutant.

<u>2. siRNA and plasmid transfection</u>

RIG-I siRNA #1 (siRNA ID #: s223615, 5' GAAGCAGUAUUUAGGGAAAtt 3'), RIG-I siRNA #2 (siRNA ID #: s24144, 5' CCAGAAUUAUCCCAACCGAtt 3') and BST2 siRNA (siRNA ID #: s2103, 5' GGAAUUCUGGUGCUCCUCAtt 3') are Silencer® Select Predesigned (inventoried) siRNAs from Ambion Life Technologies (Thermo Fisher Scientific, MA, USA). Silencer® Negative Control #1 (scramble) siRNA, and *Silencer*™ Cy™3-labeled Negative Control #1 siRNA (Catalog number: AM4621) were also purchased from Ambion Life Technologies (Thermo Fisher Scientific, MA, USA). RPAP3 siRNA was custom designed (5' GAAGGAUGUUCUGUCGAATT 3') from Ambion Life Technologies (Thermo Fisher Scientific, MA, USA). RIG-I siRNA #3 (SASI_Hs01_00047986/DDX58, 5' CCAUUGAAAGUUGGGAUUUtt 3') is predesigned (inventoried) and was purchased from MilliporeSigma, MO, USA.

All plasmids contained an insert in a pCG10-MCS vector. Full length RIG-I plasmid used a pEF-BOS vector. Lipofectamine 2000 (Thermo Fisher Scientific, MA, USA) was used as a transfection reagent. The manufacturer's recommended protocol was followed. siRNA:transfection reagent complexes were formed in Gibco™ OPTI-MEM™ Reduced Serum Medium (Thermo Fisher Scientific, MA, USA) for 20 minutes then added dropwise to cells cultured in DMEM + 10% FBS.

3. Immunofluorescence

Cells were seeded onto sterile coverslips placed in 6-well plates and cultured for 24 hours at 37°C. At the indicated timepoint, media was aspirated and the cells were washed once with PBS. The coverslips were fixed with 4% paraformaldehyde for 15 minutes at room temperature, followed by a 3X PBS wash for five minutes, then permeabilized with 0.1% Triton™ X-100 for 15 minutes at room temperature. Mouse anti-measles matrix protein (Catalog number: MAB8910, purchased from MilliporeSigma, MO, USA) was diluted 1:100 in antibody dilution buffer containing PBS + 1% bovine serum albumin (BSA) + 0.3% Triton™ X-100, then 150 µl volume was pipetted onto parafilm wax wrapped around a 96-well lid. The coverslip was then placed on the buffer and sandwiched with another layer of parafilm wax and incubated overnight at 4°C. The coverslips were then transferred back to a 6-well plate and incubated (in the dark with agitation) for two hours in 500 µl antibody dilution buffer containing anti-mouse secondary antibody 594 (1:1000) (Aliquot gifted from Dr. Luc Sabourin, Ottawa Hospital Research Institute, Ottawa, Canada) and Phalloidin-iFluor 488 Reagent (1:1000) (Catalog number: ab176753, Abcam, Cambridge, United Kingdom). Coverslips were then mounted onto microscopy slides with 15 µl Prolong™ Gold antifade reagent with DAPI to visualize nuclei (Thermo Fisher Scientific, MA, USA). Microscopy slides were imaged with a Zeiss Axioskop 2 Fluorescence Microscope (Carl Zeiss AG, Oberkochen, Germany).

<u>4. Quantifying syncytial size</u>

Nuclei were stained in two ways; in cell culture supplemented with Hoechst stain (Aliquot gifted from Dr. Rebecca Auer, Ottawa Hospital Research Institute) at a 1:400 dilution for 30 minutes, or on fixed microscopy slides with DAPI-containing mounting medium (Prolong™ Gold antifade reagent with DAPI, Thermo Fisher Scientific, MA, USA). Cell culture plates containing Hoechst stain were analyzed under the AMG EVOS® FL microscope (Thermo Fisher Scientific, MA, USA), and fixed DAPI-treated microscopy slides under the Zeiss Axioskop 2 Fluorescence Microscope (Carl Zeiss AG, Oberkochen, Germany). 40X magnification was used to identify syncytia (considered here to be any multinucleated cell with 5 or more nuclei) and the number of nuclei were manually counted. Care was taken to scan the field as not to count the same nuclei or syncytia twice. A large sample size (n = 30, or 50) was used for high statistical power. Violin plots were created using GraphPad Prism 7, and the built-in analysis software was used to perform a one-way ANOVA with Tukey's correction for multiple comparisons using a family-wise significance of p = 0.05.

5. Western blot

For sample collection, the media was first aspirated and the cells were washed with PBS. Lysates were collected using Piece™ RIPA Buffer (Thermo Fisher Scientific, MA, USA) supplemented with protease inhibitors and 10 µL/mL EDTA (Halt™ Protease Inhibitor Single-Use Cocktail (100X), Thermo Fisher Scientific, MA, USA). Protein samples were purified from the lysate by centrifugation at 18500 g for 15 minutes at 4°C. The supernatant (containing protein) was saved, and the pellet (containing DNA and cell debris) was discarded. Protein concentrations were measured by BCA assay (#23225, Pierce™ BCA Protein Assay Kit, Thermo Fisher Scientific, MA, USA). 10 µg lysates were prepared in RIPA buffer, 4X Laemmli Sample Buffer (Catalog number: 161-0747, Bio-rad Laboratories, CA, USA), and 10X DTT (0.5 M) then the samples were heated at 95°C for five minutes to denature proteins. The lysates were electrophoresed in NuPAGE™ 4-12% Bis-Tris 10-well premade gels (#NP0335BOX, Thermo Fisher Scientific, MA, USA) for one hour at 100V, then transferred to a 0.45 µm nitrocellulose membrane (Amersham™ Protran™, GE Healthcare, IL, USA) for one hour at 25V. Membranes were blocked in 5% dry milk powder dissolved in tris-buffered saline (TBS) containing 0.5% Tween 20 for one to three hours at room temperature. The membrane was rinsed with TBS-T (0.5% Tween 20). Rabbit anti-RIG-I C-terminus antibody (Catalog number: 06-1041, MilliporeSigma, MO, USA) was diluted 1:1000 in BSA and incubated with agitation overnight at 4°C. After 3X TBS-T washes, anti-rabbit IgG, HRP-linked secondary antibody (#7074, Cell Signaling Technologies, MA, USA) was diluted 1:5000 in BSA and incubated for one hour at room temperature. After 3X TBS-T washes, anti-GAPDH antibody (#2118S, Cell Signaling Technologies, MA, USA) was diluted 1:10000 in BSA and incubated for one hour at room temperature. The membrane was washed again 3X in TBS-T, then incubated in 1 mL chemiluminescent substrate (#34577, SuperSignal™ West Pico PLUS Chemiluminescent Substrate, Thermo Fisher Scientific, MA, USA). Membranes were imaged with a Bio-Rad ChemiDoc™ Imager (Bio-Rad Laboratories, CA, USA).

6. RT-PCR and RNA Sequencing

To collect RNA samples, the media was first aspirated and the cells were washed with PBS. 350 µl buffer RLT (from the RNeasy® Plus Mini Kit, Qiagen, Hilden, Germany) was supplemented with 2-mercaptoethanol and added to each well of the 6-well plate. The lysates were homogenized with QIAshredder spin columns (Qiagen, Hilden, Germany) following the manufacturer's protocol. RNA was isolated from the homogenized lysates thereafter using the RNeasy® Plus Mini Kit (Qiagen, Hilden, Germany). RNA sequencing samples were also collected in this way. For RT-PCR experiments, cDNA synthesis was performed with Superscript® III First Strand cDNA synthesis kit (Thermo Fisher Scientific, MA, USA). OneTaq DNA polymerase (New England Biolabs, MA, USA) was used for PCR amplification, following the manufacturer's protocol and adjusting melting temperatures and cDNA template amounts as needed. Primer pair sequences used for semi-quantitative RT-PCR; RIG-I: forward (5' AGA CCC TGG ACC CTA CCT AC 3') and reverse (5' GGC ATT CTG GAT CTT CTT GG 3'). β-actin: forward (5' TGG ACA TCC GCA AAG ACC TGT ACG 3') and reverse (5' CTA GAA GCA TTT GCG GTG GAC 3'). IFN-β: forward (5' GAC GCC GCA TTG ACC ATC TA 3') and reverse (5' CCT TAG GAT TTC CAC TCT GAC T 3'). MeV nucleoprotein (N): forward (5' CCA CAC TTG AGT CCT

TGA TGA ACC 3') and reverse (5' GCA GTG TCA ATG TCT AGG GGT 3'). MeV fusion glycoprotein (*F*): forward (5' AAT GCC TTC TAC CCG ARG AGT CCT 3') and reverse (5' TAT TGT TCG GCC AGA GGG AAG 3'). MeV haemagglutinin glycoprotein (*H*): forward (5' CTT CCA GGG TTG AAC ATG CTG TG 3') and reverse (5' TTA TTC TGA TGT CTA TTT CAC ACT 3'). Myoglobin (*MB*): forward (5' GAG AGA GCG GGG TCT GAT CT 3') and reverse (5' ACA GCC AGT TTG GAG GTT GG 3'). Actin related protein 2/3 complex subunit 5 (*ARPC5*): forward (5' CAC CAA GAG TCA GGC AGT GA 3') and reverse (5' AGC AGC AAG TGC CTT TTC AT 3'). Annexin A8 (*ANXA8*): forward (5' AGC ATC AAG AGT GAG ACC CA 3') and reverse (5' CGG TTG GGA TGG ATT CGT GT 3'). *YbeY*: forward (5' CAC GGA CTC TGT CAC TTG CT 3') and reverse (5' TCC CGC TTT CAG AAG GAA CG 3').

<u>7. Cloning and Site-directed Mutagenesis</u>

For cloning the exon 4 splice variant into a pCG-10 multiple cloning site (MCS) plasmid, the vector was digested with MluI-HF restriction enzyme for 15 minutes at 37°C, and blunt ends were created using the blunting enzymes and protocol from the CloneJET PCR Cloning Kit at 70°C for five minutes. (Thermo Fisher Scientific, MA, USA). The vector was dephosphorylated using the Quick Dephosphorylation Kit (New England Biolabs, MA, USA) at 37°C for 30 minutes, followed by inactivation at 80°C for two minutes. The insert was phosphorylated with the T4 Polynucleotide Kinase (Thermo Fisher Scientific, MA, USA) and adenosine triphosphate (ATP) at 37°C for 30 minutes followed by inactivation at 75°C for 15 minutes. Ligation was completed with the T4 DNA Ligase and protocol from the Rapid DNA Dephos & Ligation Kit (MilliporeSigma, MA, USA) at room temperature for 30 minutes, which was then used to transform NEB 10-beta Competent *E.coli* (High

Efficiency) (New England Biolabs, MA, USA) following the manufacturer's protocol. The next day, colonies containing the exon 4 splice variant insert in the correct orientation were identified with a single colony PCR using a gene-specific forward primer and vector-specific reverse primer. QIAprep® Spin Miniprep Kit (Qiagen, Hilden, Germany) was used for plasmid isolation from mini cultures.

To correct the RIG-I R7C SNP in the novel exon 4 splice variant, the following primer pair was used for site-directed mutagenesis of the plasmid: forward (5' GAC CAC CGA GCA GCG ACG CAG CCT GC 3') and reverse (5' GCA GGC TGC GTC GCT GCT CGG TGG TC 3'). To generate three non-synonymous mutations in the siRNA #2 binding site of RIG-I, the following primer pair was used for site-directed mutagenesis: forward (5' CCA GAA TTT AAA ACC AGA ATT ATC CCT ACA GAC ATC ATT TCT GAT CTG TCT GAA TGT TT 3') and reverse (5' AAA CAT TCA GAC AGA TCA GAA ATG ATG TCT GTA GGG ATA ATT CTG GTT TTA AAT TCT GG 3'). Q5 High-Fidelity DNA polymerase (New England Biolabs, MA, USA) was used to amplify the mutated product from 20 ng of plasmid by PCR. The QIAquick PCR Purification Kit (Qiagen, Hilden, Germany) was then used to purify the DNA. 1 µl of the purified mutant plasmid was transformed into NEB 10-beta Competent *E.coli* (High Efficiency) (New England BioLabs) following the manufacturer's protocol, mini-prepped the following day (#27106, QIAprep® Spin Miniprep Kit, Qiagen, Hilden, Germany), then sequenced to confirm their identity. Successful constructs were then maxi-prepped (#12263, QIAfilter™ Plasmid Maxi Kit) to produce high yield transfection-grade plasmids.

8. Virus titration

Three wells (biological replicates) were used for each experimental group. At the indicated time points, the supernatant was collected and saved (released fraction), and fresh pre-warmed media was replaced onto the cells. The cells were then scraped into the fresh media and collected in separate tubes (cell-associated fraction). All tubes were briefly vortexed then flash-frozen in EtOH with dry ice with and stored at -80°C overnight. After thawing, the tubes were aggressively vortexed (3X five seconds) to liberate virus particles from the cell debris, which was then pelleted at 1503 g for five minutes. Each sample was titrated in a ten-fold serial dilution four times (technical replicates) on Vero cells in a 96-well format. 48 hours later, syncytia were counted manually with the AMG EVOS® FL microscope (Thermo Fisher Scientific, MA, USA) at 2X magnification. Every sample was counted from the same column/dilution. For each biological replicate, the four technical replicates were averaged to converge on a mean value for the sample, then the three biological replicates were averaged to determine the virus concentration in cell infection units (CIU)/mL for each experimental group.

9. Cytotoxicity Assays

Each experimental group was represented by three wells (biological replicates). At the indicated time point, media was aspirated from the 12-well plate and replaced with 250 µl XTT reagent (Colorimetric Cell Viability Kit III (XTT), PromoCell) and incubated at 37°C for one hour. 75 µl of the XTT reagent was transferred into a 96-well plate times three times for each sample (technical replicates). The cells were then washed with PBS and replaced with approximately 500 µl of crystal violet stain for one hour with agitation at room temperature. Meanwhile, absorbance of the XTT reagent was measured at 465 nm and 620 nm. The 465 nm absorbance value of wells containing blank XTT reagent was subtracted from the 465 nm absorbance values of all samples, then the three technical replicates were averaged for each well. The biological replicates were standardized to mock-treated cells (considered to be 100% metabolically active) which was then averaged for the mean value of each experimental group. Once the incubation of crystal violet was complete, the stain was appropriately discarded and the wells were rinsed thoroughly with water to remove excess stain. The plate was then imaged with an Epson Perfection V600 Photo scanner.

Results

<u>1. Identification of an enhanced MeV spread phenotype</u>

To find suitable antiviral restriction factors to target with MeV-encoded amiRNAs, candidate genes were first screened with siRNA transfection prior to MeV Id-EGFP infection. Three candidate antiviral genes were selected from the literature based on their demonstration of MeV inhibition. The first target is RIG-I, the most upstream component of the interferon response to RNA viruses including MeV. Though expressed at low levels in uninfected cells, it becomes highly induced upon MeV infection, likely as a positive feedback loop to amplify the interferon response (Figure 1A). Furthermore, RIG-I is known to be crucial for interfering with MeV replication.[95] In cells deficient of RIG-I through CRISPR-Cas9 knockout, it is clear MeV infection is unrestricted (Figure 1B).

The second target is tetherin/bone marrow stromal cell antigen 2 (BST2). Tetherin/BST2 is a membrane-bound protein that tethers budding virus particles to the cell surface, thereby restricting their release and dissemination. Recently, it was found to restrict morbillivirus cell-cell fusion and replication by targeting the viral glycoproteins.[96] Specifically, MeV H protein expression is decreased in BST2-overexpressing cells, which impairs cell-cell fusion and cell-associated virus titers. The study lacked knockdown experiments, but it is reasonable to hypothesize BST2 suppression would enhance MeV spread and cytotoxicity. In two medium-resistance cancer cells, BST2 was silenced with an siRNA before infection with MeV Id-EGFP and there was no apparent difference in MeV spread compared to the scramble siRNA control group (Figure 1C). The third and last candidate is RNA polymerase II associated protein 3 (RPAP3), a subunit of the R2TP complex which co-chaperones heat shock protein 90.[97] The R2TP complex was shown to directly interact with the mumps virus (MuV) polymerase, and RPAP3 knockdown enhances MuV RNA synthesis without affecting viral replication.[98] RPAP3 knockdown similarly increases MeV RNA synthesis, but MeV replication was also enhanced. Two intermediate-resistance cancer cell lines were transfected with an RPAP3 siRNA prior to incubation with MeV Id-EGFP, and this did not promote a visible change in change in infection (Figure 1C). It should be noted that this assessment is purely qualitative by visually comparing MeV-EGFP cytopathic effects with fluorescence microscopy and quantitative conclusions have not been drawn. Furthermore, knockdown of BST2 and RPAP3 was not validated.

Intriguingly, enhanced MeV syncytial formation was identified through siRNA-mediated knockdown of RIG-I in the same two intermediate-resistance cancer cell lines, however, this phenotype was only seen with one of two RIG-I siRNAs (Figure 1D). Initially, the outcome of enhanced MeV infection was not entirely surprising given the well-established role of RIG-I in innate immunity. To quantify this observation, the nuclei of MeV-infected cells transfected with RIG-I siRNAs were visualized on fixed microscopy slides mounted in DAPI-containing medium (Figure 1E). The number of nuclei per syncytium was then manually counted with fluorescence microscopy under a 40X objective. A total of 50 syncytia (n=50) were quantified per slide, with a syncytium considered any multinucleated cell containing five or more nuclei (Figure 1F). This definition is arbitrary, with previous publications using thresholds as low as three nuclei/syncytium.[99] It is clear there are large MeV syncytia produced from pre-treatment with RIG-I siRNA #2, and this effect can be seen in other cancer cell lines from different tumour entities (Figure 1G, Table 1). Consequently, enhanced cell-cell fusion causes MeV to spread rapidly through cell monolayers *in vitro*. With live cell imaging analysis (IncuCyte Live-Cell Analysis System, Sartorius AG, Göttingen, Germany), the total GFP area of siRNA #2-transfected and MeV Id-EGFP-infected wells was accurately quantified over the course of infection (Figure 1H). Notably, the total GFP area of the well rises at a steeper rate and plateaus approximately 24 hours sooner with siRNA #2 compared to siRNA #1 and controls, implying MeV Id-EGFP is spreading at a faster rate.

Strong	Weak	Absent
U-2 OS	A549	HCT-15
PC-3	SK-MEL-2	SK-MEL-28
U-87 MG	SK-OV-3	SW620
MCF7	HT-29	Vero
		M14

Table 1: Cell line responsiveness to siRNA #2 treatment. Subjective assessment of the sensitivity of different cancer cell lines to the cell-cell fusion phenotype induced by siRNA #2. Judgments are based on fluorescent microscopy experiments of MeV Id-EGFP infection in the given cell line following siRNA #2 transfection. Fluorescent syncytia in the siRNA #2 sample were compared to siRNA #1 and scramble control.

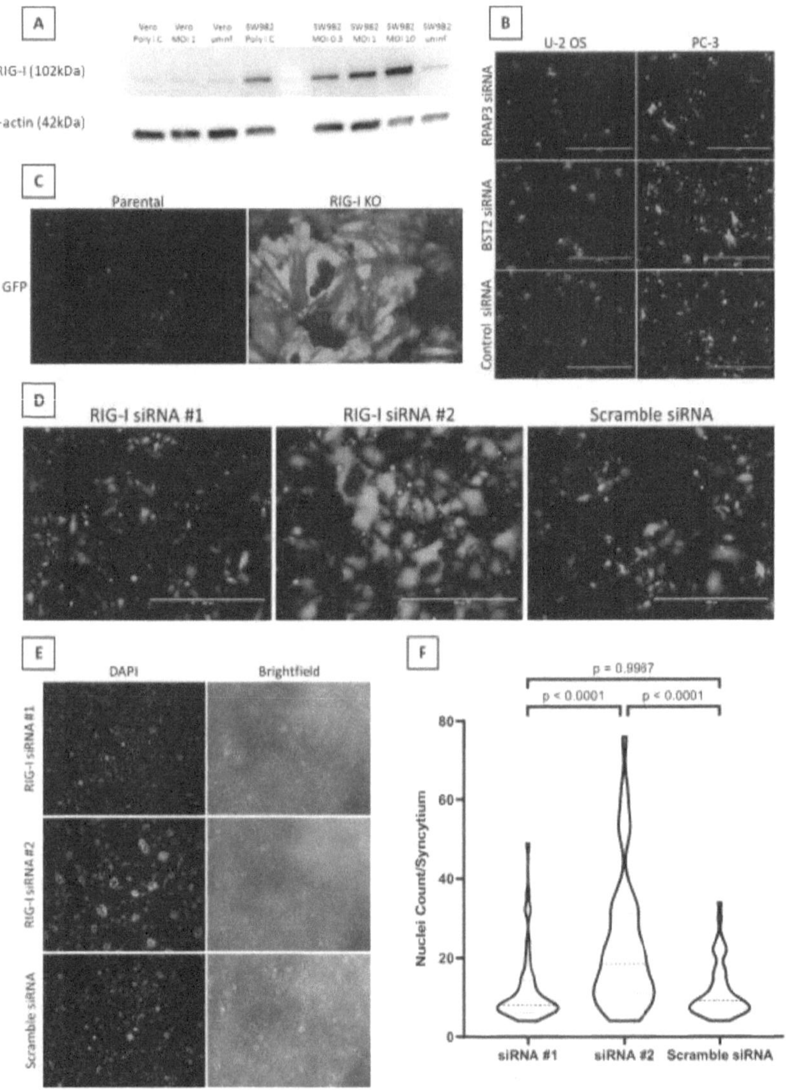

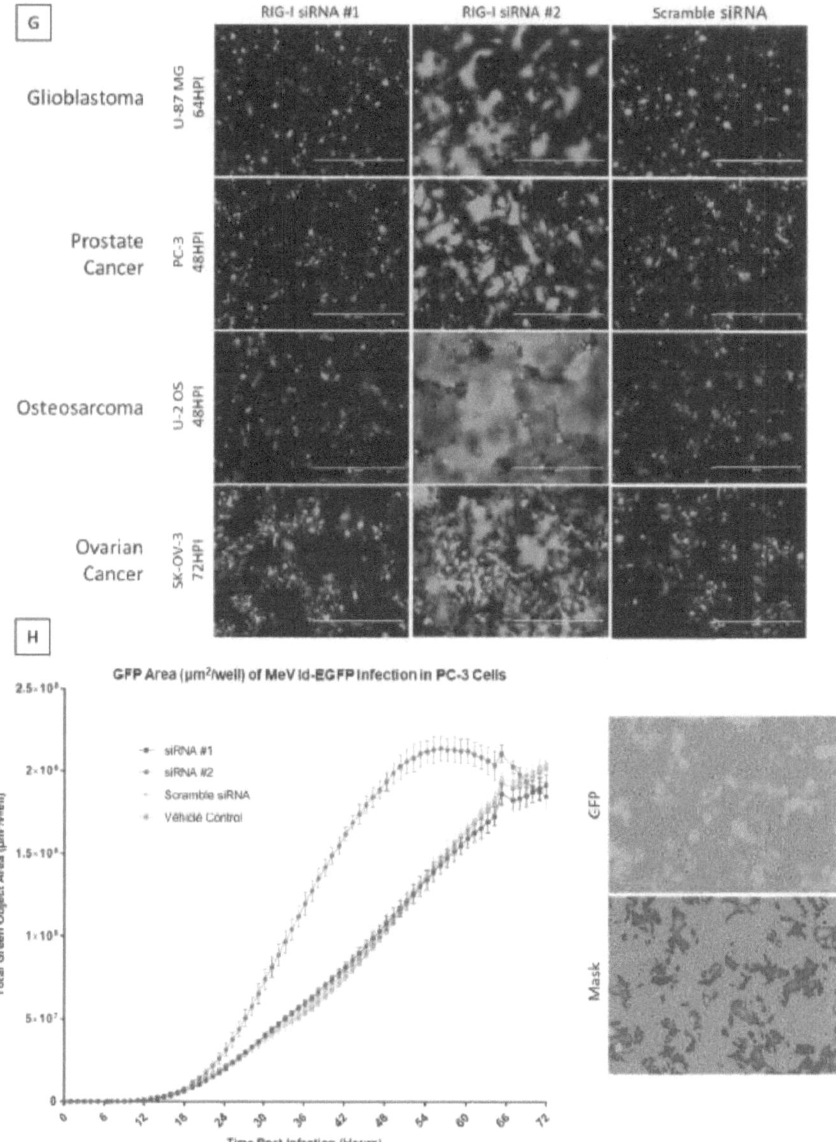

G
RIG-I siRNA #1
RIG-I siRNA #2
Scramble siRNA
Glioblastoma
U-87 MG
64HPI
Prostate
Cancer
PC-3
48HPI
Osteosarcoma
U-2 OS
48HPI
Ovarian
Cancer
SK-OV-3
72HPI
H
GFP Area (µm²/well) of MeV Id-EGFP Infection in PC-3 Cells
2.5×10⁸
2×10⁸
1.5×10⁸
1×10⁸
5×10⁷
0
Total Green Object Area (µm²/Well)
siRNA #1
siRNA #2
Scramble siRNA
Vehicle Control
0
6
12
18
24
30
36
42
48
54
60
66
72
Time Post Infection (Hours)
GFP
Mask

Figure 1: Identification of an enhanced MeV spread phenotype with RIG-I siRNA #2.
(A) Vero (African green monkey kidney epithelial cells) and SW982 (synovial sarcoma cells) lysates were blotted for RIG-I expression. PolyI:C was included as a positive control for RIG-I activation. Vero cells served as a negative control due to an impaired interferon response. Escalating virus concentrations correlate with RIG-I expression in SW982 cells, indicative of RIG-I upregulation upon infection. **(B)** U-2 OS and PC-3 cancer cell lines, infected with MeV Id-EGFP MOI 0.01. GFP images were captured at 48hpi. Cells were transfected with 20nM siRNA targeting the corresponding genes prior to infection. **(C)** Fluorescence microscopy images of A549 RIG-I $^{-/-}$ and parental cells infected with MeV NSe Id-EGFP (MOI 0.03) at 48hpi. Both cell lines were pretreated with a Cy3-labelled non-targeting siRNA control. **(D)** PC-3 cells infected with MeV Id-EGFP at 36hpi after 10nM siRNA transfection. **(E)** U-87 MG cells infected with MeV Id-EGFP (MOI 0.1) for 48h after 20nM siRNA transfection. Microscopy slides were fixed in 4% paraformaldehyde and mounted in DAPI-containing mounting medium. Both DAPI and brightfield images were captured under a 10X objective. **(F)** Nuclei/syncytium violin plots. With the same slides in Figure E, the number of nuclei in 50 syncytia (n=50, at least 5 nuclei/syncytium) were quantified under a 40X objective. A one-way analysis of variance (ANOVA) reached statistical significance, which was followed by a post hoc test using Tukey's method. P values for the comparisons between all groups are shown. **(G)** Screening RIG-I siRNA #2 in various cancer cell lines. Cells were transfected with 20nM siRNAs and infected with MeV Id-EGFP (MOI 0.03). GFP images were captured at the indicated time points. **(H)** Live cell imaging analysis (IncuCyte Live-Cell Analysis Systems). PC-3 cells were infected with MeV Id-EGFP (MOI 0.03) and GFP images were captured every hour for 72h. A mask was built (representative images on the right) to accurately quantify GFP signal area. Total GFP area of the well was measured with the software and plotted against time. N = 3 wells were tested for each group, with the average plotted +/- SEM.

2. Preliminary assay validation

siRNA #2 clearly enhances MeV infection, but it is interesting how siRNA #1 did not have the same effect. siRNA #1 and #2 both target RIG-I, so their phenotype should theoretically be the same. It could be that siRNA #1 is somehow dysfunctional. To gain insight into this, siRNA transfection efficiency and RIG-I knockdown were validated in PC-3 prostate cancer cells. A fluorescently-labelled siRNA was chosen to assess siRNA transfection efficiency in this cell line. PC-3 cells were imaged six hours post transfection (HPTR) with a Cy3-labelled non-targeting siRNA which confirmed these cells internalize the siRNAs efficiently (Figure 2A). In the same experiment, target knockdown was measured at the RNA and protein levels by semi-quantitative RT-PCR and western blot respectively. The HDAC-inhibitor suberoylanilide hydroxamic acid (SAHA) was naively introduced with the intention of blocking interferon production as a positive control. SAHA was previously shown to reduce interferon alpha (IFN-α) expression in PC-3 cells infected with VSV.[100] However, preliminary testing with MeV had not been performed, and 5 µM SAHA had no apparent effect on MeV infection (Figure 2B). Furthermore, there is no rational for SAHA or dimethyl sulfoxide (DMSO) affecting RIG-I expression so this should be overlooked when interpreting the target knockdown validation experiments. At 36 HPI, lysates were tested for RIG-I expression at the protein (Figure 2C) and RNA (Figure 2D) level, both of which indicated siRNA #1 and #2 are functional. These early results were intriguing because there are strikingly different phenotypes between the two siRNAs that downregulate the same target.

Since RIG-I is upstream in the interferon response, it is possible the downstream integrity of the pathway differs. To this end, interferon beta (IFN-β) expression was roughly evaluated by semi-quantitative RT-PCR in unsaturated conditions, where fainter bands are seen with both siRNA #1 and #2 compared to the controls (Figure 2E). Taken together, these initial experiments suggest both RIG-I siRNAs are functioning similarly to suppress the interferon pathway, which raises the suspicion that the identified phenotype is specific to siRNA #2 and independent of RIG-I suppression.

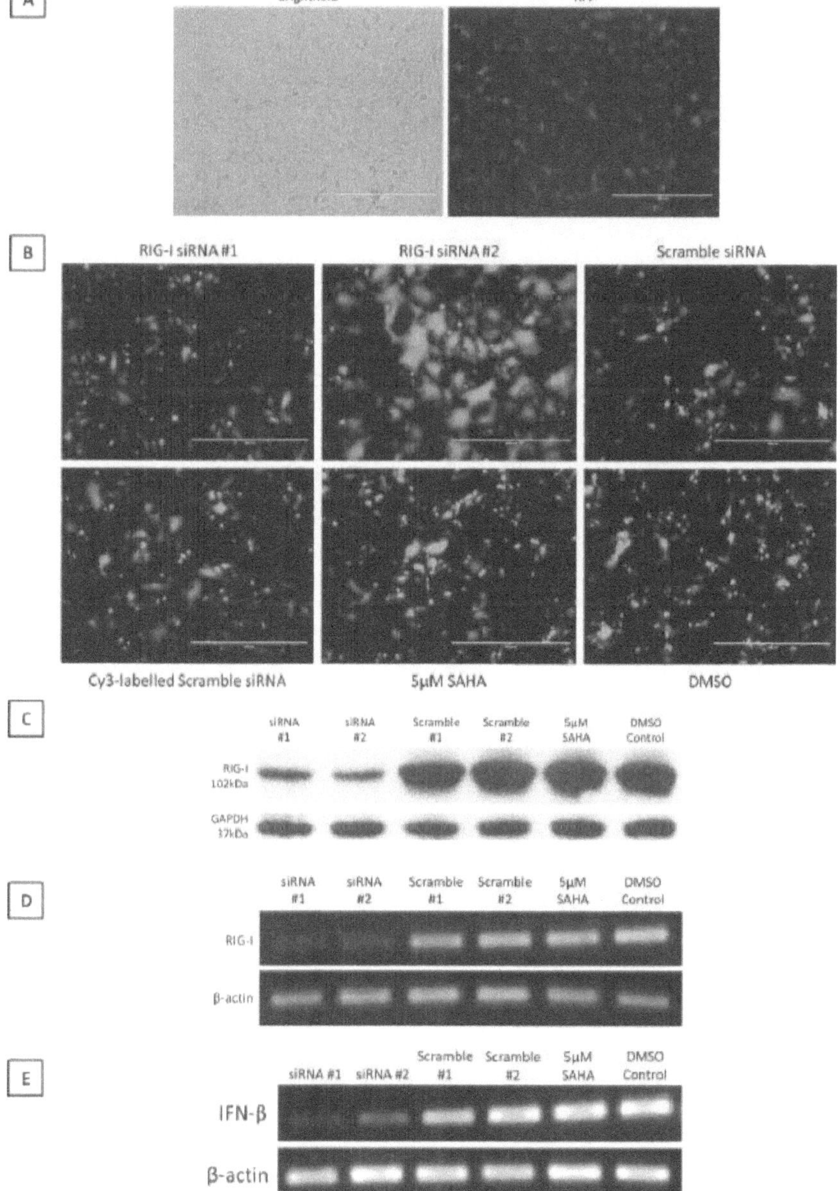

A
Brightfield
RFP
B
RIG-I siRNA #1
RIG-I siRNA #2
Scramble siRNA
Cy3-labelled Scramble siRNA
5µM SAHA
DMSO
C
siRNA #1
siRNA #2
Scramble #1
Scramble #2
5µM SAHA
DMSO Control
RIG-I 102kDa
GAPDH 37kDa
D
siRNA #1
siRNA #2
Scramble #1
Scramble #2
5µM SAHA
DMSO Control
RIG-I
β-actin
E
siRNA #1
siRNA #2
Scramble #1
Scramble #2
5µM SAHA
DMSO Control
IFN-β
β-actin

Figure 2: Validating transfection efficiency and target knockdown with RIG-I siRNA #1 and #2. All data in this figure was collected from the same experiment. PC-3 cells were transfected with 10 nM siRNAs for 6 hours, or treated with 5 µM of SAHA (or DMSO control), followed by infection with MeV ld-EGFP (MOI 0.01). **(A)** At 6 HPTR, brightfield and RFP images were captured from the Cy3-labelled scramble siRNA group after a PBS wash to validate siRNA internalization. **(B)** GFP images of the infection were captured at 36 HPI. **(C)** At 36 HPI, lysates were harvested and a RIG-I western blot was performed to confirm RIG-I knockdown with the siRNAs. **(D)** RIG-I semi-quantitative RT-PCR of cDNAs from lysates collected at 36 HPI. 20 ng (RIG-I) and 10 ng (β-actin) cDNA template was PCR amplified for 30 cycles. Four repetition experiments with the same cDNA samples gave identical results where both siRNA #1 and #2 suppress IFN-β expression. **(E)** Semiquantitative RT-PCR for IFN-β expression in siRNA-transfected and MeV-infected PC-3 cell cDNA samples. Data is representative of three independent experiments. 20 ng (IFN-β) and 10ng (β-actin) was amplified for 30 cycles with gene-specific primers. In figures C-E, Scramble #1 is the non-labelled scramble siRNA and Scramble #2 is the Cy3-labelled scramble siRNA.

<u>3. Identification of a novel RIG-I splice variant</u>

To explain how two functional siRNAs could yield different phenotypes, three hypotheses were developed and tested; *(1)* there could be different RIG-I isoforms that are differentially targeted, *(2)* the position of the siRNA target site at either the N- or C-terminus is somehow relevant, and *(3)* there is unintended downregulation of another gene with siRNA #2.

The isoform hypothesis is based on the concept that there are RIG-I splice variants (SV) with differential functions, and perhaps one exists which is missing the siRNA #2 target site from alternative splicing. Specifically, it would be a RIG-I exon three splice variant, since the target site for siRNA #2 is in this exon. In this case, full-length wildtype RIG-I would be downregulated by siRNA #2, but the exon three splice variant would be unaffected (Figure 3A). Furthermore, the variant could be functional, since many RIG-I mutants have dominant negative properties.[93] Dominant negative mutants are alternatively spliced or otherwise mutated variants of a gene that have antagonistic characteristics.[101] This idea is also supported by a dominant negative RIG-I splice variant missing exon two, which is proximal to the siRNA #2 target site.[102] PCR amplification of the RIG-I tandem CARDs (exons 1-5) yielded a major band as expected, but also a faint minor band (Figure 3B) that was initially predicted to be the exon two splice variant. However, gel extraction and sequencing revealed this minor band is an uncharacterized exon four splice variant. Since the nucleotide length of exon four is not divisible by three, the splicing event induces a downstream frameshift which creates a premature stop codon immediately after the splice site (Figure 3C). Therefore, this novel RIG-I isoform would likely produce a truncated protein encoding exons 1-3. Since siRNA #2 targets exon three, the exon four splice variant would also be suppressed, therefore it would be unrelated to the cell-cell fusion phenotype.

This uncharacterized isoform encodes the complete first CARD and part of the second CARD of RIG-I. Truncated RIG-I constructs which encode the tandem CARDs (exons 1-5) cause constitutive signalling, although the complete tandem is needed for this activity.[93] Constructs encoding either CARD alone fail to signal IFN-β promoter induction and lack dominant negative activity.[93] Nevertheless, the exon four splice variant was cloned for further study into its potential functions.

The best follow-up experiment would be a western blot to detect this variant at the protein level, but this was not possible with our antibody raised to C-terminal epitopes. Therefore, an overexpression study was initiated to address its role in MeV infection. Due to its weak expression in PC-3 and HEK 293T cells, different cell lines were screened for higher expression of the splice variant by RT-PCR (Figure 3D). Lysates from MeV-infected HCT-15 cells yield a particularly strong minor band, so this sample was selected for gel extraction. Sequencing results revealed an R7C single nucleotide polymorphism (SNP) in the splice variant (Figure 3E). This is a common mutation which partially inactivates RIG-I and leads to its overexpression, which explains the appearance of strong bands amplified from HCT-15 lysates.[103] The R7C mutation was corrected by site-directed mutagenesis and cloned into a eukaryotic expression vector. A full-length RIG-I plasmid was obtained from Dr. Carolina Ilkow (Ottawa Hospital Research Institute, Ottawa, Canada) as a positive control. Overexpression of the exon four SV was found to have no effect on MeV Id-EGFP infection compared to the empty vector (Figure 3F). On the other hand, RIG-I overexpression inhibits the virus as expected. This suggests the

SV is non-functional, or at least it does not have a meaningful influence on MeV infection. This endogenous RIG-I SV is being reported for the first time, but without further investigation, it is believed this SV is a candidate for nonsense mediated decay. Exploration of potential RIG-I splice variants involving any of exons two through four has given no indication of an isoform involved in the siRNA #2-induced fusion phenomenon, thereby rejecting the isoform hypothesis. Interestingly, the dominant negative exon two splice variant was never detected in these experiments.

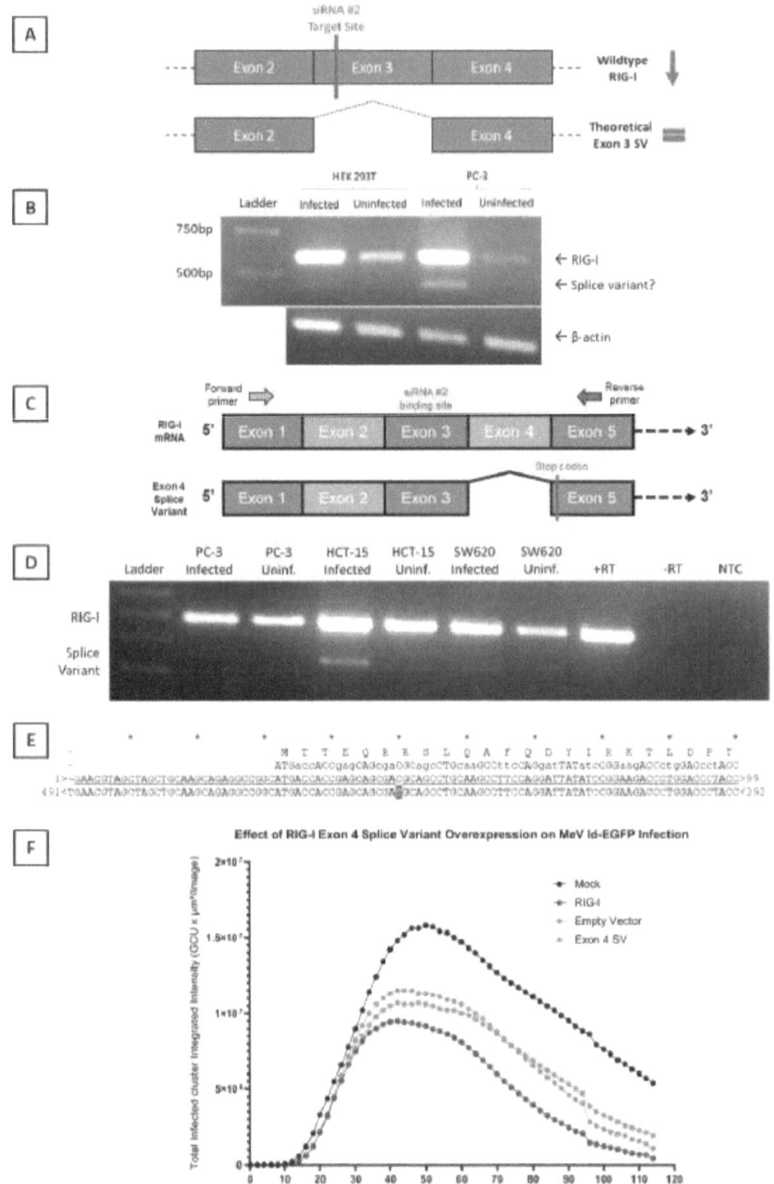
A
siRNA #2 Target Site
Exon 2
Exon 3
Exon 4
Wildtype RIG-I
Exon 2
Exon 4
Theoretical Exon 3 SV
B
HEK 293T
PC-3
Ladder
Infected
Uninfected
Infected
Uninfected
750bp
500bp
RIG-I
Splice variant?
β-actin
C
Forward primer
siRNA #2 binding site
Reverse primer
RIG-I mRNA
5'
Exon 1
Exon 2
Exon 3
Exon 4
Exon 5
3'
Exon 4 Splice Variant
Stop codon
5'
Exon 1
Exon 2
Exon 3
Exon 5
3'
D
Ladder
PC-3 Infected
PC-3 Uninf.
HCT-15 Infected
HCT-15 Uninf.
SW620 Infected
SW620 Uninf.
+RT
-RT
NTC
RIG-I
Splice Variant
E
M T T E Q R R S L Q A F Q D Y I R E T L D P T
F
Effect of RIG-I Exon 4 Splice Variant Overexpression on MeV Id-EGFP Infection
Total Infected cluster Integrated Intensity (GCU x µm²/image)
Mock
RIG-I
Empty Vector
Exon 4 SV
Elapsed Time (Hours)

Figure 3: Identification of a novel exon four RIG-I splice variant. (A) Schematic of the RIG-I isoform hypothesis. The siRNA #2 target site is in exon three of RIG-I which downregulates wildtype RIG-I. A theoretical exon three splice variant would avoid knockdown. **(B)** RT-PCR amplification of RIG-I exons 1-5 in PC-3 and HEK 293T cell lysates (infected versus uninfected). Major band is full length RIG-I, minor band is a RIG-I splice variant. **(C)** Schematic of the novel RIG-I exon four splice variant, with a premature stop codon after the splice site. **(D)** Screening different cancer cell lysates (infected with MeV versus uninfected) for strong RIG-I exon four splice variant expression by RT-PCR with the exon 1-5 primer pair. **(E)** Sequencing analysis of the gel-extracted RIG-I exon four splice variant. The SV sequencing file was aligned to full length wildtype RIG-I (accession number: NM_014314.4). The highlighted thymine nucleotide misaligns with wildtype RIG-I, and this SNP causes a nonsynonymous R7C point mutation. The top sequence is wildtype RIG-I and the bottom sequence is the exon four splice variant. **(F)** Live cell imaging analysis (IncuCyte) of RIG-I exon four SV overexpression on MeV Id-EGFP infection. The RIG-I exon four splice variant was cloned and overexpressed in A549 cells. An empty vector pCG-10 MCS plasmid (negative control) and full-length RIG-I plasmid (positive control) were included to compare the effects of the SV on MeV infection. 500 ng of the indicated plasmid was transfected for 24 hours prior to infection. The mock control is un-transfected. Cells were infected with MeV-Id-EGFP (MOI 0.1) and GFP images were captured every two hours for 114 hours. A mask was built to accurately quantify GFP area and intensity, which was then plotted against time. One replicate was used for each group.

4. The enhanced MeV spread phenotype is specifically induced by siRNA #2

The second hypothesis is related to the isoform hypothesis in that the location of the siRNA target site along the RIG-I transcript is important. siRNA #1 and #2 target opposite ends of the RIG-I transcript, specifically exons 16 and three respectively. To determine if the phenotype is caused by targeting this specific region in exon three, a third RIG-I siRNA was ordered with its target site positioned immediately next to that of siRNA #2 (Figure 4A). Another advantage to this experiment is having a third siRNA specific to RIG-I. If the fusion phenotype is only present after transfection with one of three RIG-I siRNAs, it further supports the hypothesis of an off-target effect. Transfection of siRNA #3 did not yield the same effect on MeV as siRNA #2 (Figure 4B), despite suppressing RIG-I at both the RNA (Figure 4C) and protein level (Figure 4D). Likewise, IFN-β expression was partially suppressed with all three siRNAs (Figure 4E). Furthermore, since the target site of siRNA #3 resides in exon three, the same as siRNA #2, these results support the conclusion that RIG-I isoforms are not involved in the enhanced MeV spread phenotype. With there being three functional RIG-I siRNAs, and only one giving a unique phenotype, there is a greater likelihood it is caused by a sequence-dependent siRNA off-target effect.

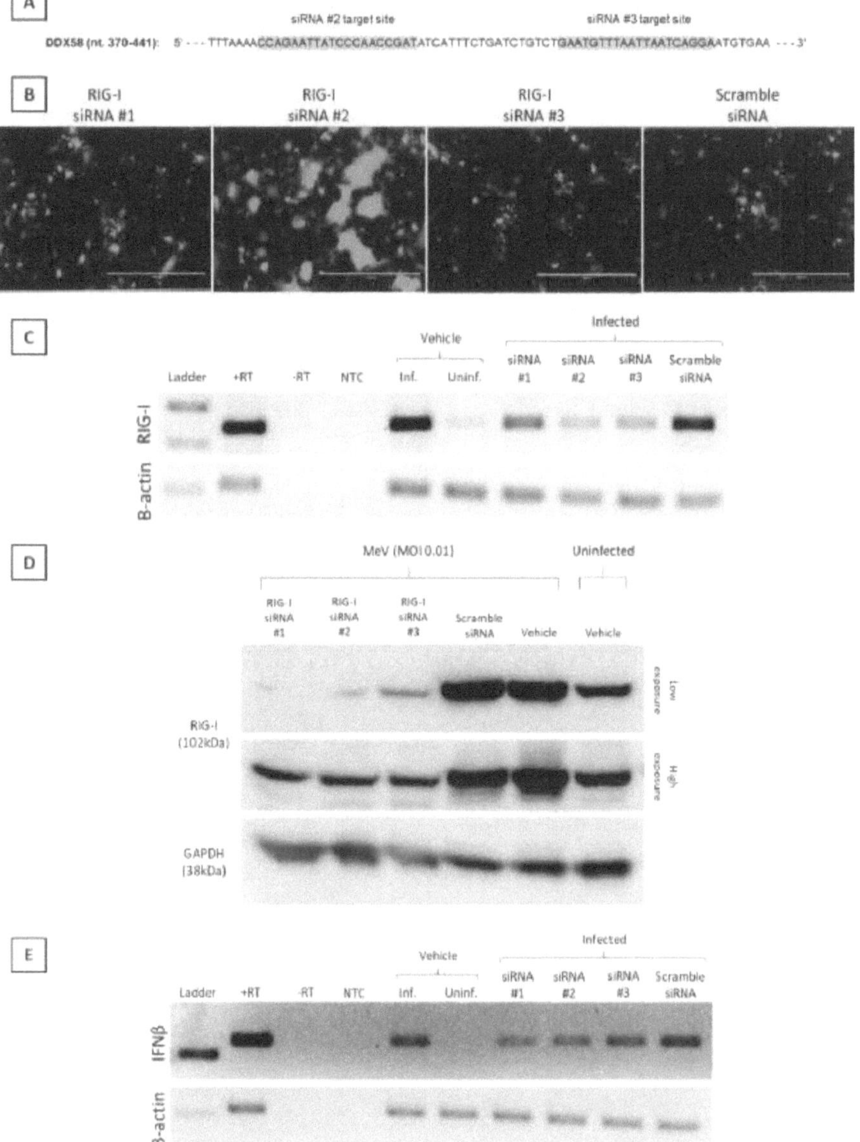

A
siRNA #2 target site
siRNA #3 target site
DDX58 (nt. 370-441): 5' - - - TTTAAAACCAGAATTATCCCAACCGATATCATTTCTGATCTGTCTGAATGTTTAATTAATCAGGAATGTGAA - - - 3'
B
RIG-I siRNA #1
RIG-I siRNA #2
RIG-I siRNA #3
Scramble siRNA
C
Vehicle
Infected
Ladder +RT -RT NTC Inf. Uninf. siRNA #1 siRNA #2 siRNA #3 Scramble siRNA
RIG-I
B-actin
D
MeV (MOI 0.01)
Uninfected
RIG-I siRNA #1
RIG-I siRNA #2
RIG-I siRNA #3
Scramble siRNA
Vehicle
Vehicle
RIG-I (102kDa)
Low exposure
High exposure
GAPDH (38kDa)
E
Vehicle
Infected
Ladder +RT -RT NTC Inf. Uninf. siRNA #1 siRNA #2 siRNA #3 Scramble siRNA
IFNβ
B-actin

Figure 4: RIG-I knockdown is not sufficient to induce the enhanced spread phenotype after MeV infection. All lysates were collected from the same experiment. **(A)** Schematic of siRNA #2 and siRNA #3 target sites in the third exon of RIG-I. **(B)** GFP images of MeV infection after transfection with three different RIG-I siRNAs, including siRNA #3. PC-3 cells were infected with MeV Id-EGFP (MOI 0.03) after 20 nM siRNA transfection and GFP images were captured at 72 HPI. Notably the phenotype is only present with siRNA #2. **(C)** Semi-quantitative RT-PCR of RIG-I expression from PC-3 cell lysates at 40 HPI. 20 ng of cDNA template was PCR amplified for 30 cycles with both the RIG-I and β-actin primer pairs. Data is representative of two repetitions with the same cDNA samples. **(D)** RIG-I western blot to assess target knockdown. MeV-infected PC-3 cell lysates (MOI 0.01) were collected at 40 HPI and blotted with RIG-I and GAPDH antibodies. Low and high exposures are presented. **(E)** Semi-quantitative RT-PCR of IFN-β expression in PC-3 cells at 40 HPI. 4 ng of cDNA template was PCR amplified for 28 cycles with IFNβ and β-actin primer pairs.

siRNA off-target effects can be reduced by using low siRNA concentrations that are still sufficient to downregulate the target.[104] In a serial dilution assay of siRNA #2, the fusion phenotype was not present below 10 nM, despite RIG-I suppression observed at 1 nM (Figure 5A, Figure 5B). Importantly, this experiment set a threshold concentration of 10 nM siRNA #2 to induce the phenotype. With this information, a serial dilution assay of siRNA #2 and #3 was performed using higher siRNA concentrations, in case a high siRNA #3 concentration is needed to induce the phenotype. As well, it is important to see if there is a dose response with siRNA #2, where a greater effect might be seen with higher concentrations. The observable threshold was again seen at around 10 nM siRNA #2, but there was no further enhancement of MeV fusion with escalating concentrations of siRNA #2 (Figure 5C). This suggests the phenotype is triggered like an on-off switch, and afterwards the effect is not dose dependent. It could be that these high siRNA concentrations do not cause further knockdown after 10 nM, because it appears RIG-I suppression is present at 1 nM siRNA concentration but plateaus at 10 nM (Figure 5D). This is consistent with a report of siRNA on-target suppression, as well as off-target gene deregulation due to competition with the endogenous RNAi machinery, reaching a maximal dose response at 20 nM.[105]

The second piece of information is that siRNA #3 does not produce the same effect as siRNA #2, even at high siRNA concentrations. Though lacking a supplementary RIG-I western blot to track expression dynamics, attempts were made to prohibit MeV spread induced with siRNA #2 by overexpressing RIG-I in conjunction with siRNA transfection. In these preliminary experiments, siRNA #2 still enhances MeV cell-cell fusion in the presence of RIG-I overexpression (Figure 5E).

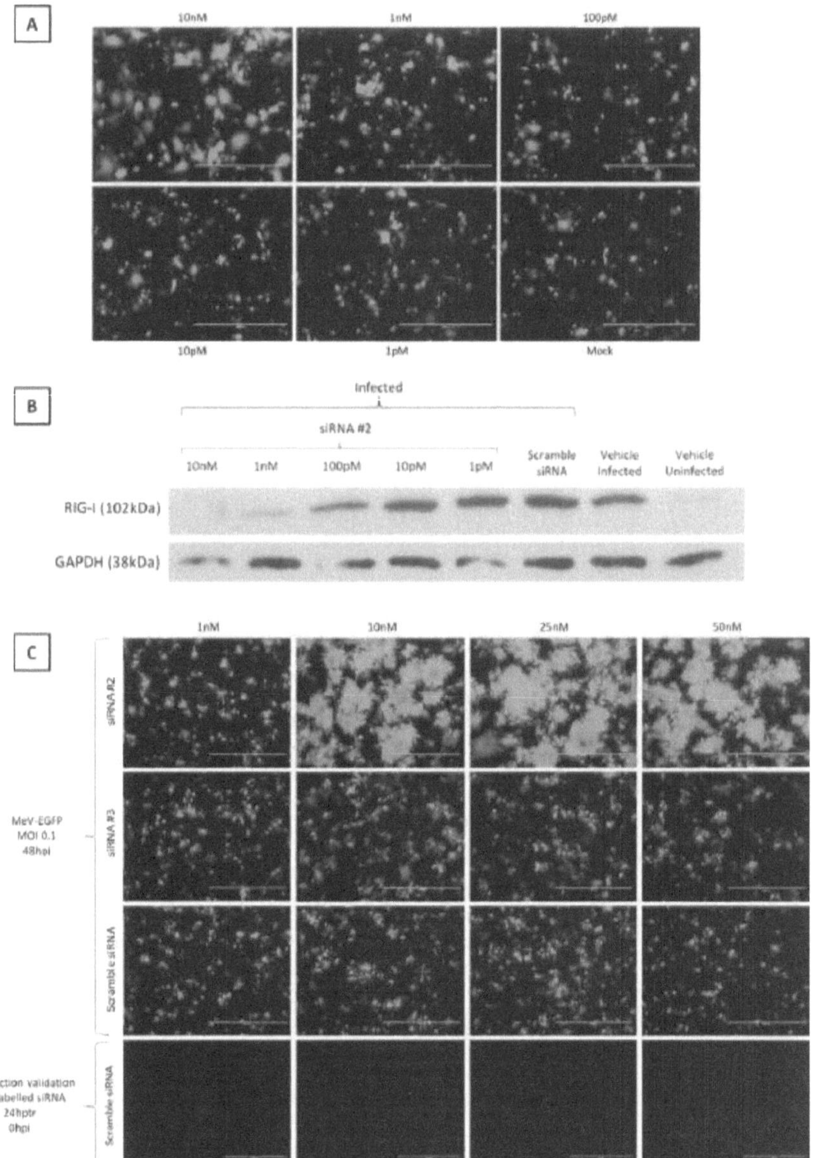
A
10nM
1nM
100pM
10pM
1pM
Mock
B
Infected
siRNA #2
10nM
1nM
100pM
10pM
1pM
Scramble siRNA
Vehicle Infected
Vehicle Uninfected
RIG-I (102kDa)
GAPDH (38kDa)
C
1nM
10nM
25nM
50nM
siRNA #2
siRNA #3
Scramble siRNA
Scramble siRNA
MeV-EGFP
MOI 0.1
48hpi
Transfection validation
Cy3-labelled siRNA
24hptr
0hpi

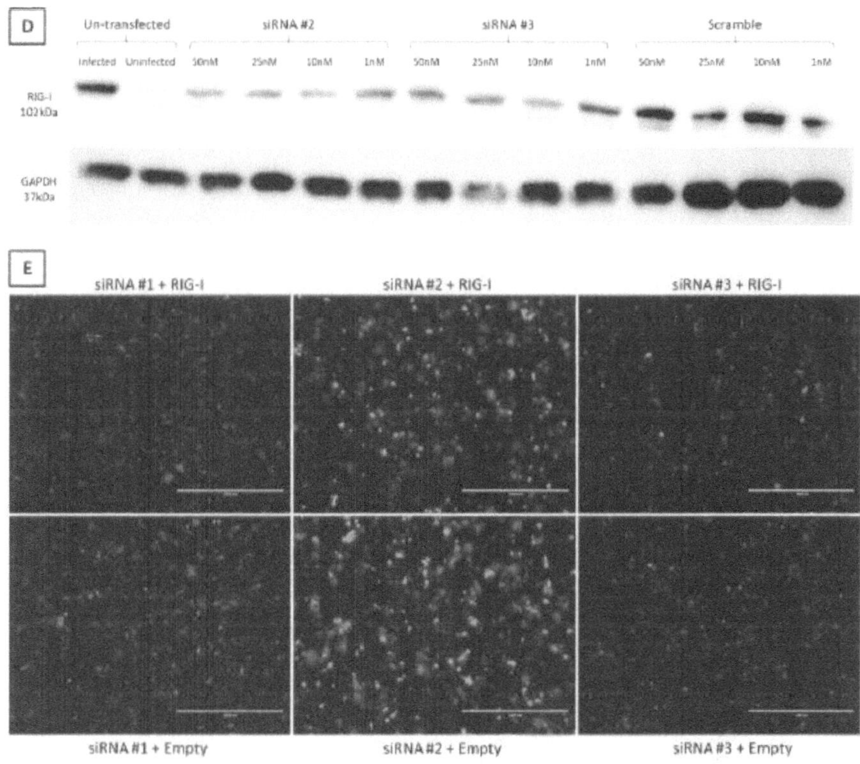

Figure 5: Serial dilution assay and dose response to RIG-I siRNA #2. (A) Ten-fold serial dilution assay of siRNA #2 starting at the highest concentration of 10 nM. GFP images of MeV Id-EGFP-infected (MOI 0.01) PC-3 cells were captured at 48 HPI. **(B)** Lysates were collected at 48 HPI, and a RIG-I western blot confirmed target knockdown at siRNA concentrations below 10nM. **(C)** Serial dilution of siRNA #2 and #3 using siRNA higher concentrations than (B) in U-2 OS cells. GFP images were captured at 48 HPI with MeV Id-EGFP (MOI 0.1). RFP images of the Cy3-labelled scramble siRNA control were included to show the extent of siRNA transfection 6 HPTR after a PBS wash. **(D)** RIG-I western blot confirming target knockdown in the siRNA #2 and #3 serial dilution assay. Lysates were collected at 48 HPI for analysis. **(E)** GFP images of MeV Id-EGFP infection in PC-3 cells at 48 HPI following a six-hour co-transfection of 300 ng plasmid and 20 nM siRNA.

Typically, viral cytopathic effects correlate with virus replication, especially when considering the role of RIG-I in antiviral signalling. However, initial titration experiments measuring the total amount of virus particles (cell associated and released) showed no difference in virus production from siRNA #2 despite the presence of large syncytia (Figure 6A). These results were surprising at first, however multiple experiments in different cell lines with varied protocols gave similar results. Serendipitously, the supernatants from siRNA #2 and scramble control samples were saved from a previous western blot experiment, and the released virus concentrations were measured with a TCID50 protocol. A near ten-fold decrease in MeV was detected in the supernatant of siRNA #2 compared to the scramble control (Figure 6B). To then better assess the differences between the cell-associated and released particles, the two fractions were harvested separately for virus titration at 60 HPI. Again, less viral particles were detected in the supernatants of siRNA #2-treated cells, but the amount of virus in the cell-associated fraction remained constant (Figure 6C). The ratio of released virus to total virus is small, which could explain why no differences in total virus was initially detected. A multi-step growth curve examined viral replication kinetics over time (Figure 6D). 24 HPI is considered early in MeV infection, and there appears to be a delay in cell-associated virus production with siRNA #2. However, at 48- and 72 HPI, which are considered intermediate and late stages of MeV infection, there is no difference between siRNA #1 and #2 in the lysates but a ten-fold difference in the supernatant. By comparing siRNA #1 and #2, there is no correlation between virus replication and cell-cell fusion, and budding into the supernatant seems to be impaired by siRNA #2.

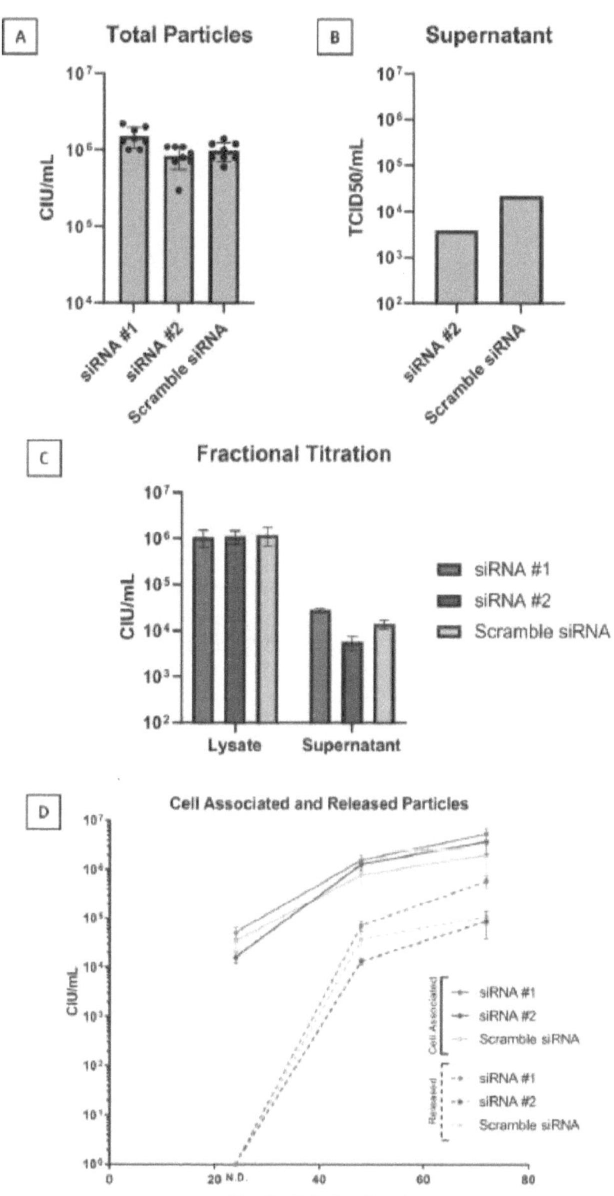
A
Total Particles
CIU/mL
siRNA #1
siRNA #2
Scramble siRNA
B
Supernatant
TCID50/mL
siRNA #2
Scramble siRNA
C
Fractional Titration
CIU/mL
Lysate
Supernatant
siRNA #1
siRNA #2
Scramble siRNA
D
Cell Associated and Released Particles
CIU/mL
Time Post Infection (Hours)
Cell Associated
siRNA #1
siRNA #2
Scramble siRNA
Released
siRNA #1
siRNA #2
Scramble siRNA
N.D.

Figure 6: siRNA #2 reduces virus detected in the supernatant but does not affect MeV replication. (A) Quantifying total virus production in MeV-infected PC-3 cells at 30 HPI following transfection with RIG-I siRNA #1 and #2. The intended MOI was 0.03, but microscopy images suggest the MOI was inadvertently higher. Total virus was harvested by scraping the cells into their supernatant. Each condition is represented by one well. Virus was quantified by counting syncytia from a serial dilution of the sample. Syncytia were counted from the same column for all samples. Each sample was measured with eight technical replicates, indicated by a single data point on the graph. **(B)** Quantifying virus in the supernatant of MeV-infected U-2 OS cells (MOI 0.1) transfected with siRNA #2 or scramble control. Each condition is represented by one well, where the supernatant was collected and virus was measured by TCID50 on Vero cells. **(C)** Quantifying MeV in cell lysates and the supernatant separately. U-2 OS cells were infected with MeV (MOI 0.03) for 60 hours after transfection with RIG-I siRNA #1 and #2. The media was removed (released particles) and the cells were scraped into fresh media (cell-associated particles) and all samples were flash frozen. After thawing, the samples were serially diluted (ten-fold) and syncytia were counted. Each condition was performed in triplicate (n=3). Each sample was measured four times to converge on the mean for that replicate. The three replicates were averaged to converge on the mean for that condition +/- SD. **(D)** Multi-step growth curve (MOI 0.1) of viral replication kinetics in U-2 OS cells. Samples were treated, prepared, and measured as in (C) at 24-, 48-, and 72 HPI. Data points are the average of three wells per sample, with each well being measured four times. The growth curve is representative of two independent experiments. CIU: Cell infectious units.

6. The mechanism does not influence MeV fusion machinery

Since there is no correlation between syncytia size and virus replication, the viral components responsible for cell-cell fusion (the F and H envelope glycoproteins) were studied more closely. First, MeV fusion (F) and haemagglutinin (H) expression was quantified at the RNA level by semi-quantitative PCR from MeV-infected lysates of cells that had been transfected with RIG-I siRNA #1 and #2 (Figure 7A). There is a small and reproducible increase in MeV F expression, but results with MeV H have been variable. Without available F and H antibodies, their expression at the protein level could not be tested, so current conclusions are based solely on RNA expression. ^{35}S radioisotope labelling reveals the active translation rates of all proteins inside the cell including the viral proteins. There is host translational shutdown with siRNA #2 at 48 HPI, but it is not clear if this is underlying the fusion phenotype, or if it is a result of more cells becoming infected by advanced MeV spread (Figure 7B). MeV is known to induce translational shutoff, so culturing the cells in a fusion inhibitor peptide (FIP) could address this uncertainty.[106] Viral protein bands are clearly seen after 48 HPI, and their intensities are indifferent across the samples. This implies there is no difference in the amount of viral proteins actively translated at this time.

Other possibilities which could promote MeV cell-cell fusion include greater entry receptor (CD46, CD150/SLAMF1, PVRL/nectin-4) expression in siRNA #2-transfected cells, or more efficient MeV glycoprotein processing/trafficking/stability in the membrane. Since F and H are sufficient to induce cell-cell fusion in the absence of virus, fusion assays are used to study these proteins in isolation. and theoretically this would involve the aforementioned possibilities. siRNA #2 was co-transfected with F, H, and RFP, and showed no effect on syncytia formation in the absence of virus (Figures 7C, 7D). Since there were multiple nucleic acids delivered simultaneously, it could be that an inadequate amount of siRNA was internalized by the cells to trigger the fusion phenotype. To validate siRNA uptake, lysates were collected to probe for RIG-I knockdown (Figure 7E). RIG-I is effectively suppressed by siRNA #1 and #2, which infers they are both functional in the assay, and the lack of differential glycoprotein fusion activity is not due to poor siRNA #2 transfection. Since the fusion phenotype is only seen after transfection of siRNA #2 with MeV infection, and not transfection of its fusogenic glycoproteins, this suggests the siRNA is not acting directly on F and H.

Perhaps a component of the antiviral response is crucial to the mechanism promoting siRNA #2-induced syncytial formation, so polyinosinic:polycytidylic acid, which is a double-stranded RNA synthetic analog, was introduced into the fusion assay but interfered with transfection efficiency (data not shown). As an alternative, infection with ultraviolet irradiated virus was considered.

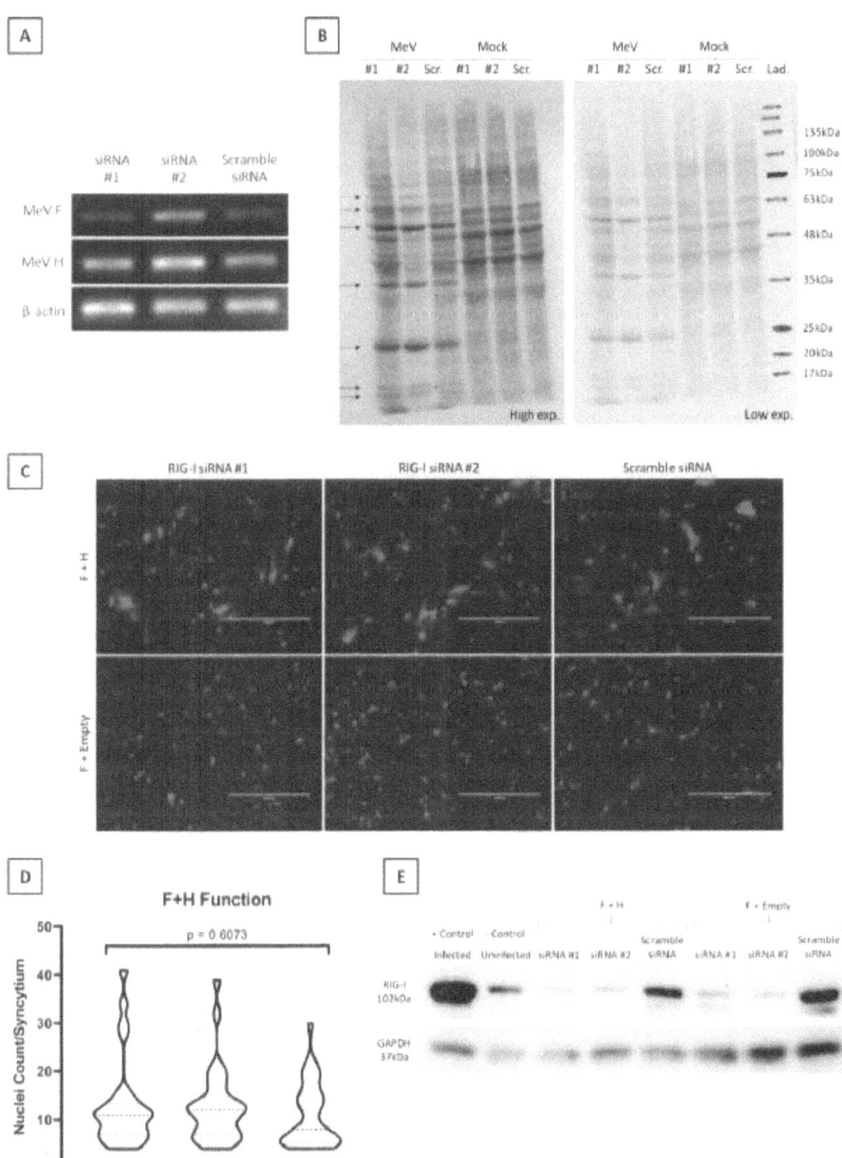

Figure 7: siRNA #2 does not affect MeV glycoproteins. (A) Semi-quantitative RT-PCR of MeV glycoprotein (F and H) expression. PC-3 cells were infected with MeV Id-EGFP (MOI 0.03) and lysates were collected after 36 HPI. 20ng of cDNA template was amplified for 30 cycles with MeV gene-specific primers (F and H) as well as β-actin. Data is representative of three independent experiments. **(B)** U-2 OS cells (infected or uninfected) were spiked with ^{35}S radionuclide at 48 HPI and lysates were exposed on film overnight. Probable MeV protein bands are indicated with black arrows. High and low exposures are shown. **(C)** Fusion assay fluorescent microscopy images including RIG-I siRNA #1 and #2. 100 ng of RFP (to better visualize syncytia and transfection efficiency), MeV F, and MeV H or empty vector plasmids were co-transfected with 20 nM of RIG-I siRNAs. A Cy3-labelled scramble siRNA was included to confirm siRNA transfection efficiency (data not shown). F + empty serves as a negative control. RFP images were captured 42 HPTR. The images shown are representative of two independent experiments. **(D)** The same fusion assay protocol was followed in a separate experiment, and Hoechst's stain was added to the media at 66 HPTR to visualize nuclei. The amount of nuclei/syncytium was quantified for 30 syncytia (n=30, where a syncytium contains at least 5 nuclei) by manually counting under high magnification. One-way ANOVA fails to reach statistical significance (p=0.6073). **(E)** RIG-I target knockdown validation. Lysates from Figure C were collected at 42 HPTR and probed for RIG-I expression to confirm siRNA transfection.

7. Investigating MeV maturation and egress

The key conclusions are that MeV replication is mostly unaffected by the presence of siRNA #2, there is a robust decrease of viral particles in the supernatant, and the mechanism of enhanced cell-cell fusion does not directly affect the glycoproteins. Since F and H are unaffected by the siRNA, this suggests other components of the virus are involved in the mechanism causing this spread phenotype. MeV matrix protein (M) is a strong candidate, because it regulates F and H fusion activity by directly binding to their cytoplasmic tails.[46] It is also central to MeV assembly and budding, which could relate to the decrease in viral particles detected in the supernatant. Actin filament disruption impairs MeV M trafficking, and leads to identical characteristics seen with the fusion phenotype induced by siRNA #2.[53]

Immunofluorescence staining of MeV matrix protein in infected U-87 MG cells was used to study the intracellular localization of the matrix protein during the siRNA #2 spread phenotype (Figure 8A). This primarily addresses potential changes in M trafficking. In this experiment, generally, the matrix protein signal is fainter in syncytia transfected with siRNA #2 at 48 HPI, however this could be due to the large size of these multinucleated cells compared to other groups. As well, the epifluorescence microscope is suboptimal to accurately pinpoint signal localization because of spillover in the Z-axis. Confocal microscopy offers better optical resolution in the Z-plane, and it shows no significant redistribution of MeV M in the same U-87 MG microscopy slides (Figure 8B). It should be noted that the Z-plane seems to vary between the samples, which is particularly noticeable in the FITC/F-actin channel. As well, insufficient time was spent analyzing the slides with confocal microscopy, so the available data is limited.

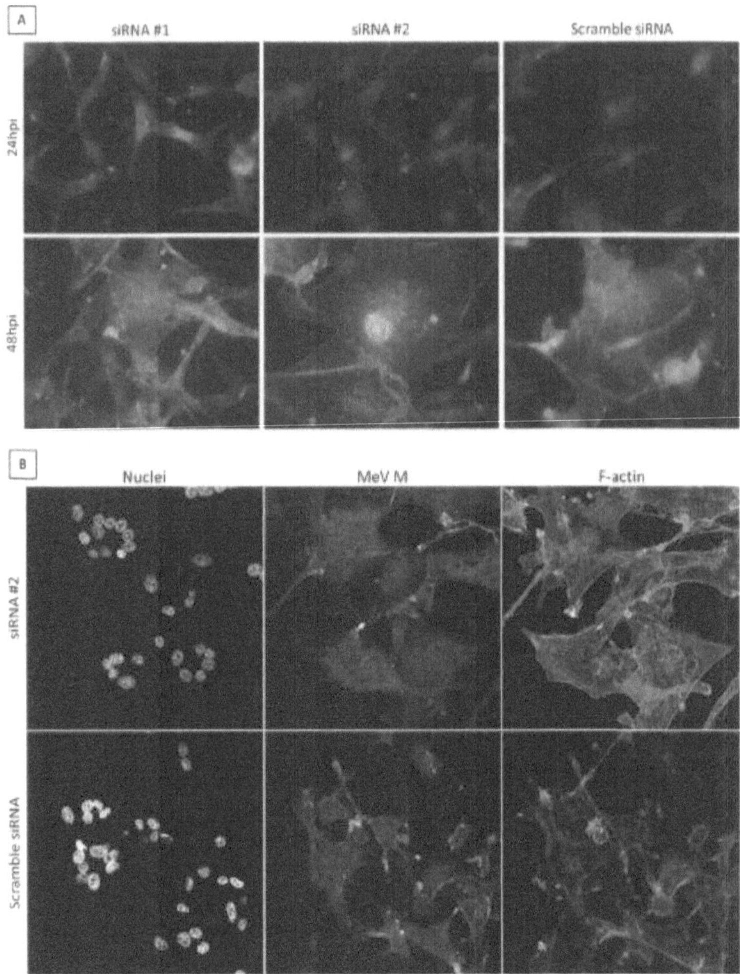

Figure 8: Investigating MeV matrix protein localization in infected siRNA #2-treated U-87 MG syncytia. (A) Immunofluorescence staining of MeV M (red) and F-actin (green) in U-87 MG cells infected at a high MOI with MeV and transfected with the corresponding siRNAs. Cells cultured and treated on cover slips were fixed at 24- and 48 HPI. A relatively small siRNA #2-transfected syncytium is represented next to average-sized siRNA #1 and control-transfected syncytia. **(B)** Confocal microscopy images of the same microscopy slides as (A). Contrast was adjusted for MeV M and F-actin images.

In follow-up experiments, syncytial size was normalized by introducing a fusion inhibitor peptide to prevent MeV-induced cell-cell fusion for a more invariable comparison between the siRNA groups. In U-2 OS cells treated with FIP, infected cells remained mononuclear after 48 HPI (Figure 9A). Within infected cells, there is no significant difference in MeV M signal intensity or localization. In the surrounding region, neighbouring cells display MeV M signal as seen in the siRNA #2-transfected sample in Figure 9A. This could be caused by cell-free virus transmission, or they could infectious-centers which are contact-dependent and differ from syncytia in that the plasma membrane is intact.[107] In either case, the size and abundance of these secondary infections appear to be indifferent between the siRNA groups. As a control, U-2 OS cells were subjected to the same siRNA and virus treatment without FIP. In this case, multinucleated cells of similar size were selected for imaging, meaning that average-sized syncytia for siRNA #1 and scramble are shown beside a relatively small siRNA #2-transfected syncytia. U-2 OS cells pretreated with siRNA #2 before MeV infection typically show fainter MeV M signal (Figure 9B). A likely explanation is that there are less cells involved in the siRNA #2 syncytia in this figure. But a clearly differentiating characteristic of large siRNA #2-transfected syncytia is a lack of nuclei and F-actin concentrating at its center. In most siRNA #1- or scramble-transfected syncytia, the nuclei are tightly clustered in the middle of the cell, whereas in the large siRNA #2-transfected syncytia, there is very little F-actin complexity in central regions and the nuclei are pulled towards the periphery (Figure 9C). This currently remains an observation in this one experiment with U-2 OS cells, but it shows an interesting variance in syncytial morphology that is likely caused by the large size of these syncytia.

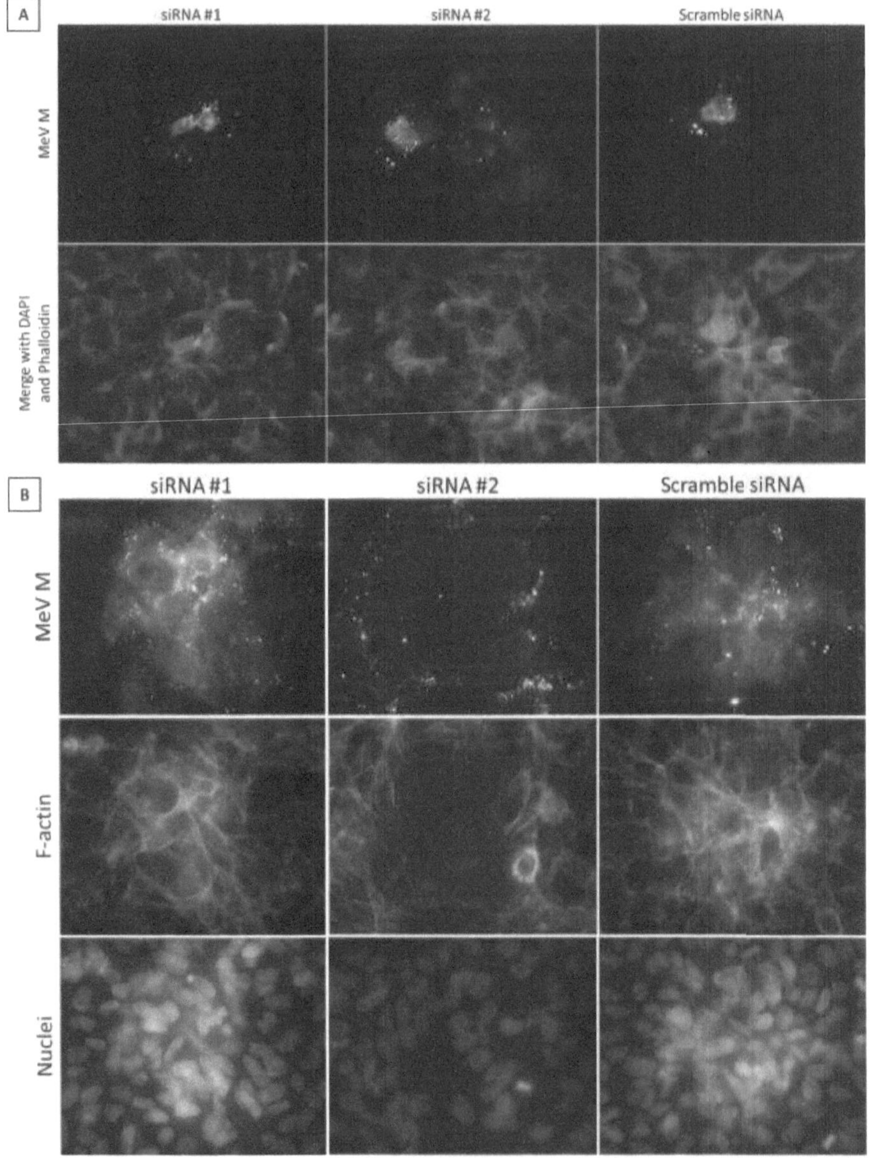

A
siRNA #1
siRNA #2
Scramble siRNA
MeV M
Merge with DAPI and Phalloidin
B
siRNA #1
siRNA #2
Scramble siRNA
MeV M
F-actin
Nuclei

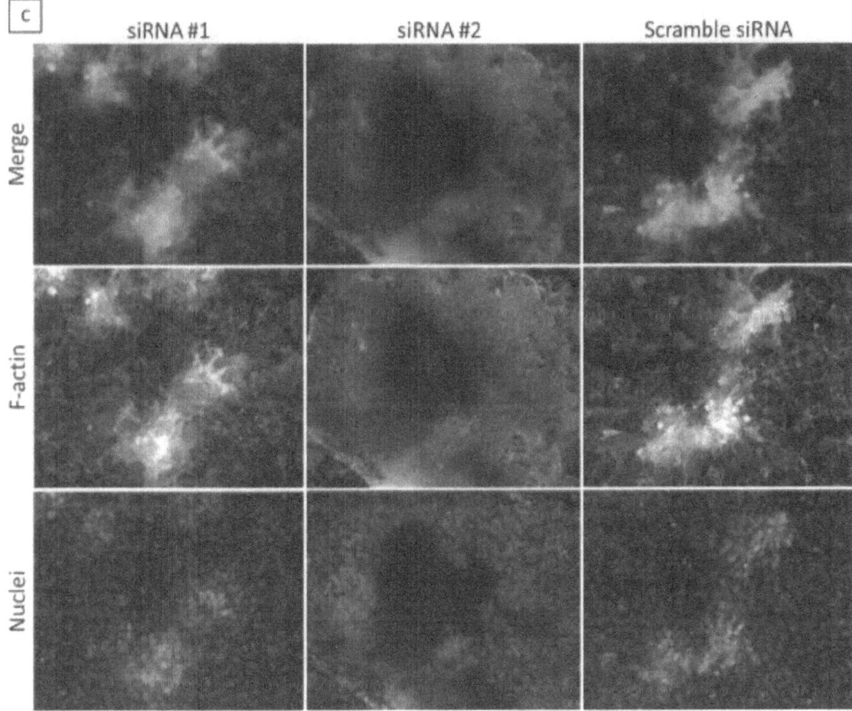

Figure 9: Investigating MeV matrix protein localization and syncytial morphology in siRNA #2-treated U-2 OS syncytia cultured in FIP. (A) Immunofluorescence staining of MeV M and F-actin in cells treated with FIP. U-2 OS cells seeded on coverslips were treated with the indicated siRNAs and infected with MeV then were cultured in FIP-containing media. The coverslips were fixed at 48 HPI, stained, then mounted in a DAPI-containing mounting medium prior to immunofluorescence microscopy. An individual isolated cell (or two) infected with MeV was identified and imaged for each condition. Images were taken under a 63X oil objective. **(B)** Immunofluorescence staining of MeV M and F-actin in multinucleated cells. These samples were treated in parallel to (A) but were not cultured in FIP to allow for MeV cell-cell fusion. Images were taken under a 63X oil objective. A small siRNA #2-transfected syncytium is shown, compared to average-sized siRNA #1- and control-transfected syncytia. **(C)** 20X oil objective images of F-actin and nuclei from the same microscopy slides shown in (D). Characteristic syncytia are shown for each condition.

During all immunofluorescence experiments, care was taken to focus on different sections of the cell, particularly the basolateral and apical membranes. This is because in polarized epithelial cells, MeV matrix protein predominantly sorts to the apical membrane.[108] Limited by poor optical resolution in the Z-plane, it is difficult to assess such patterns in trafficking. However, the bright dots seen in MeV M-stained microscopy slides are mainly found on the basolateral surface. These dots are not seen in a primary antibody control slide, and are never found in uninfected regions. Furthermore, it's seen that MeV M is less abundant, but not completely absent, from the nuclei of infected cells (Figure 8C). This supports a previous study, where MeV matrix protein has been shown to partially localize to the nucleus where it interferes with host cell transcription.[109] Nuclear MeV M localization was carefully considered, and no apparent difference is seen between the siRNA groups. Lastly, MeV M typically colocalizes with F-actin, which is not a particularly novel observation, but this interaction is independent of treatment with the siRNAs.

To summarize, there is a lack of clear evidence to conclude any difference in MeV M localization because of siRNA #2. This is in part made difficult by extreme variation in syncytial size between siRNA #2 and controls. Because there is no clear indication thus far, it seems MeV M trafficking is not impaired by siRNA #2.

8. Off-target candidate search

The most interesting explanation for the observed phenotype is siRNA-mediated off-target suppression of a gene other than RIG-I. This has been reported before, but there is not an established pipeline to identify such off-target mRNAs.[110,111] To narrow down the list of possible off-target mRNAs, the Basic Local Alignment Search Tool developed by the National Center for Biotechnology Information (NCBI BLAST) was used to find host genes that have perfect complementarity with the guide strand seed region of siRNA #2, since this is a primary determinant of off-target suppression.[87] Genes that seed-match with the passenger strand were included as well, because in some cases it can have silencing activity.[112] RNA sequencing was then performed to explore transcriptomic changes, and the reads per kilobase of transcript per million mapped reads (RPKM) analysis was cross-referenced to the list of seed-matched off-target candidates. Theoretically, both siRNA #1 and #2 should have an identical expression profile since both siRNAs target RIG-I, and any outliers could be indicative of the mechanism promoting MeV syncytium formation. A549 cells were selected based on previous characterization of their response to siRNA #2-enhanced MeV spread (Figure 10A). These cells were infected with MeV ld-EGFP (MOI 0.1) following transfection with siRNA #1 and #2. The fusion phenotype was weak, but present at 48 HPI (Figure 10B). Tables 2A and 2B show separate RPKM analyses of seed-matched genes by two independent collaborators.

	Gene Name	siRNA #1 + MeV	siRNA #2 + MeV	Fold Change
Guide Strand	DDX58	155.639	168.029	0.93
	MB	14.91	6.22	2.39
	YBEY	38.20	26.76	1.43
	CIDEB	1.96	1.37	1.42
	CHURC1	84.4356	62.403	1.35
	RILPL2	5.53	5.12	1.08
	LRRC61	1.37	1.29	1.06
	ANXA8L1	53.61	52.22	1.03
	PLPPR4	1.12685	1.2086	0.93
	ANXA8	25.59	28.66	0.89
	NOP9	20.1207	31.9377	0.63
	ADCY10			
	DNAH2			
Passenger Strand	ARPC5	167.00	18.80	8.88
	FTL	10865.2	3834.22	2.83
	ELMO1	10.6542	4.3664	2.44
	LGALS4	2.45555	1.65248	1.49
	GPATCH1	4.27786	3.08994	1.38
	AMACR	21.1782	15.6462	1.35
	EHD4	37.6507	31.084	1.21
	AMBRA1	44.2115	36.7993	1.20
	VAMP7	36.3364	30.4979	1.19
	ZNF420	8.07721	7.30539	1.11
	FXYD6	20.2405	18.4776	1.10
	WDR81	11.0198	10.1266	1.09
	SNX14	90.7457	84.7999	1.07
	RAB24	35.1645	33.5533	1.05
	ZNF461	7.70448	7.48724	1.03
	RAD50	51.8805	51.1827	1.01
	HCAR2	5.40397	5.37928	1.00
	MSANTD4	25.5535	25.5822	1.00
	KIAA0232	21.1452	21.3721	0.99
	ACVR1	43.2487	43.8489	0.99
	INPP5A	14.4988	15.1699	0.96
	SYT13	113.527	122.468	0.93
	CSE1L	122.328	134.404	0.91
	PARP9	486.638	538.627	0.90
	TLL1	7.49656	8.40046	0.89
	CEP170	34.1009	38.7592	0.88
	ETS1	15.0152	17.6463	0.85
	TRIM31	55.0235	76.9605	0.71
	DNAJC10	37.781	59.5507	0.63

Table 2A

Table 2B

	Gene Name	siRNA #1 + MeV	siRNA #2 + MeV	Fold Change
Guide Strand	DDX58	51.79	52.14	0.99
	MB	5.32	2.56	2.08
	CHURC1	31.03	21.76	1.43
	YBEY	19.10	14.26	1.34
	ANXA8L1	19.73	17.11	1.15
	RILPL2	1.45	1.35	1.07
	ANXA8	10.94	10.41	1.05
	NOP9	10.52	12.06	0.87
	CIDEB			
	LRRC61			
	PLPPR4			
	ADCY10			
	DNAH2			
Passenger Strand	FTL	4468.77	1520.97	2.94
	ELMO1	4.08	1.39	2.93
	FXYD6	13.36	8.08	1.65
	WDR81	2.83	1.85	1.53
	EHD4	13.62	10.66	1.28
	AMBRA1	15.06	11.85	1.27
	ZNF420	2.68	2.11	1.27
	RAB24	18.72	15.72	1.19
	ZNF461	5.67	4.79	1.19
	MSANTD4	6.07	5.26	1.15
	ARPC5	87.43	77.54	1.13
	SNX14	16.05	15.08	1.06
	AMACR	14.64	14.35	1.02
	ACVR1	15.07	14.96	1.01
	INPP5A	4.22	4.31	0.98
	SYT13	41.29	42.62	0.97
	GPATCH1	7.29	7.55	0.97
	HCAR2	1.56	1.65	0.95
	DNAJC10	42.25	44.52	0.95
	KIAA0232	7.69	8.29	0.93
	CSE1L	40.21	43.95	0.91
	PARP9	151.30	168.91	0.90
	TRIM31	6.96	8.26	0.84
	TLL1	2.01	2.46	0.82
	CEP170	13.24	16.58	0.80
	ETS1	4.22	5.36	0.79
	VAMP7	6.29	9.79	0.64
	RAD50	10.25	21.03	0.49
	LGALS4			

DExD/H-Box helicase 58 (*DDX58*), the gene encoding RIG-I, is shown at the top of each table. RIG-I transcript levels are near identical in the siRNA #1- and siRNA #2-transfected samples, which supports the conclusion that both siRNAs are equivalently functional at silencing RIG-I. Actin related protein 2/3 complex subunit 5 (*ARPC5*) was an attractive candidate in the first analysis (Table 2A) due to having one of the highest fold changes in the dataset, as well as perfect seed complementarity with the passenger strand of siRNA #2. ARPC5 is an integral component of the Arp2/3 complex, and interfering with ARPC5 directly inhibits Arp2/3 complex formation and function.[113] The Arp2/3 complex has a critical role in actin cytoskeleton dynamics, which as mentioned previously, influences MeV maturation and fusion. To validate the RNA sequencing results, expression of *ARPC5* was assessed in both PC-3 and A549 cells treated with siRNA #2 by semiquantitative RT-PCR (Figure 10C). There was no indication of any change in *ARCP5* RNA expression across all samples, and this could be explained by signal saturation, which was then addressed by titrating the PCR cycles. Later, a second independent RPKM analysis (Table 2B) was completed but showed *ARPC5* expression is similar between the samples, which differs from the first analysis (Table 2A). Both the RT-PCR results and secondary analysis suggest there is in fact no change in *ARPC5* expression between siRNA #1 and #2, and the large foldchange in analysis #1 is likely an erroneous outlier.

Given the apparent discrepancy in RPKM values, genes with a foldchange greater than two were compared between both data sets. The rationale is that genes which are significantly suppressed by siRNA #2 in separate analyses are more likely to be biologically true. 26 genes are commonly downregulated, three of which have perfect complementarity with the seed regions of siRNA #2. Ferritin light chain (*FTL*), and engulfment and cell motility 1 (*ELMO1*) have a perfect seed-match with the passenger strand so were included in Tables 2A and 2B. Myoglobin (*MB*), which was originally identified as a seed-matched gene from NCBI BLAST, has perfect complementarity with the guide strand.

The presence of myoglobin outside of cardiac and muscle tissues is surprising, but recent publications have shown ectopic *MB* expression in cancer driven by a novel alternative promoter.[114,115] Interestingly, in an unpublished database of the human interactome by high-throughput affinity purification-mass spectrometry, one of its few interactors is YbeY, which is another seed-matched candidate.[116] *YbeY* is a poorly characterized mitochondrial protein and was recently shown to have an essential role in mitochondrial translation and oxidative phosphorylation.[117] This is interesting because the Database for Annotation, Visualization and Integrated Discovery (DAVID) reveals mitochondrial translation, ribosomes, and cellular respiration are some of the most enriched classifications of genes suppressed more than 1.5-fold by siRNA #2.[118,119] Using available PC-3 cDNA, a preliminary RT-PCR for *MB* and *YbeY* expression confirmed ectopic *MB* expression in this cell line, as well as an indication of siRNA #2-mediated *MB* suppression (Figure 10D). cDNA was then prepared from MeV-infected and siRNA-transfected A549 cells to bridge the RT-PCR experiments and RNA sequencing results. In the A549 RT-PCR experiments, *MB* is also expressed in this lung adenocarcinoma cell line, albeit weakly, and the *MB* band is similarly faintest in the siRNA #2 group (Figure 10E). Repetition experiments were expanded using appropriate controls, and each time it appears *MB* is suppressed by siRNA #2 (Figure 10F). Also, there is some indication that *MB* is upregulated upon MeV infection, however this is currently an observation lacking rigor. Several repetition experiments with cDNAs from both cell lines indicate off-target *MB* suppression with siRNA #2, and so far, this is the only gene where this is observed consistently at the mRNA level.

Annexin A8 (*ANXA8*) is another interesting candidate, because two other members of the annexin family are known to be important in MeV maturation and fusion. Briefly, ANXA2 is the only known factor to traffic MeV M to the plasma membrane, and ANXA1 is important for MeV fusion pore expansion.[52,120] Both RPKM analyses indicate no change in *ANXA8* RNA expression between the two siRNA samples, but a preliminary RT-PCR result has shown a decrease in *ANXA8* cDNA from siRNA #2-transfected A549 cells (Figure 10G). Repetition experiments had given variable results between the siRNA groups, so robust conclusions cannot be drawn unless consistent results are seen, especially in different cell lines. However, technical replicates of the same cDNA samples have reproducibly shown an increase in *ANXA8* expression upon MeV infection.

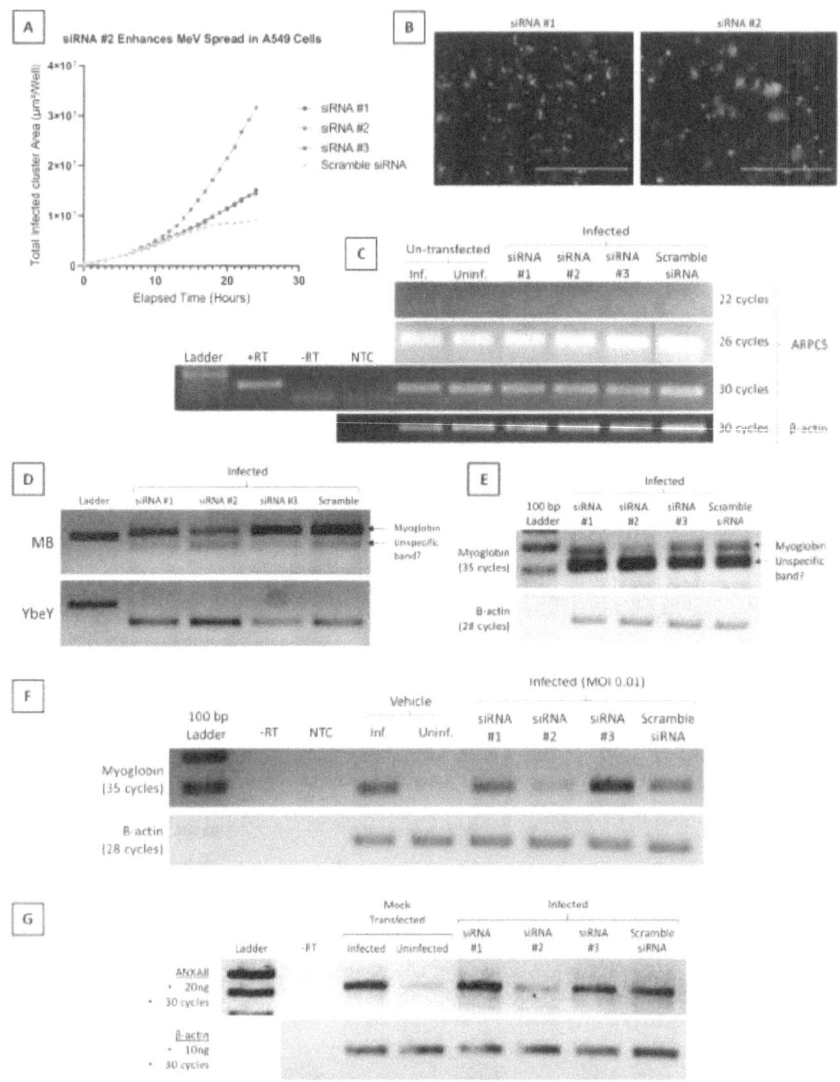
A
siRNA #2 Enhances MeV Spread in A549 Cells
Total Infected cluster Area (µm²/Well)
Elapsed Time (Hours)
siRNA #1
siRNA #2
siRNA #3
Scramble siRNA
B
siRNA #1
siRNA #2
C
Un-transfected
Infected
Inf.
Uninf.
siRNA #1
siRNA #2
siRNA #3
Scramble siRNA
22 cycles
26 cycles
ARPC5
30 cycles
30 cycles
β-actin
Ladder
+RT
-RT
NTC
D
Infected
Ladder
siRNA #1
siRNA #2
siRNA #3
Scramble
MB
Myoglobin
Unspecific band?
YbeY
E
Infected
100 bp Ladder
siRNA #1
siRNA #2
siRNA #3
Scramble siRNA
Myoglobin (35 cycles)
Myoglobin
Unspecific band?
β-actin (28 cycles)
F
Infected (MOI 0.01)
100 bp Ladder
-RT
NTC
Vehicle
Inf.
Uninf.
siRNA #1
siRNA #2
siRNA #3
Scramble siRNA
Myoglobin (35 cycles)
β-actin (28 cycles)
G
Mock Transfected
Infected
Ladder
-RT
Infected
Uninfected
siRNA #1
siRNA #2
siRNA #3
Scramble siRNA
ANXA8
20ng
30 cycles
β-actin
10ng
30 cycles

Figure 10: Evidence of siRNA #2-mediated off-target suppression in seed-matched genes other than RIG-I. (A) IncuCyte live cell imaging analysis of MeV Id-EGFP spread in A549 cells transfected with the three RIG-I siRNAs. After siRNA transfection, A549 cells were infected with MeV Id-EGFP (MOI 0.01) and GFP images were automatically captured every hour for 24 hours. GFP area of the well was measured by the IncuCyte software and plotted against time. Each condition is represented by one replicate. **(B)** GFP images of samples prepared for RNA sequencing. A549 cells were transfected with 20 nM siRNA and infected with MeV Id-EGFP (MOI 0.1). Total RNA was harvested at 48 HPI when the images were taken. **(C)** Semi-quantitative RT-PCR for ARPC5 expression to validate RNA sequencing results. 20 ng A549 cDNA was amplified with ARPC5- or β-actin-specific primers for the indicated amount of cycles. The A549 cells were treated with the RIG-I siRNAs and infected with MeV, and RNA was isolated at 48 HPI. **(D)** Semi-quantitative RT-PCR for MB and YbeY expression in MeV-infected and siRNA-transfected lysates harvested at 40 HPI. The top band is MB, and the minor band is unknown. **(E)** Semiquantitative RT-PCR repetition for myoglobin expression with cDNA from infected and siRNA-treated A549 cells (48 HPI) to validate RNA-sequencing results. **(F)** Semi-quantitative RT-PCR for myoglobin expression from PC-3 cell lysates at 40 HPI. The bottom part of the MB gel was cropped to exclude the minor band. **(F)** Semi-quantitative RT-PCR for ANXA8 expression in cDNAs from MeV-infected and siRNA-transfected A549 cells at 48 HPI. -RT: Reverse transcriptase control. NTC: No template control.

<u>9. Greater spread leads to greater MeV cytotoxicity in cancer cell lines *in vitro*</u>

The finding that siRNA #2 promotes MeV syncytia formation is not only interesting because of its potential to uncover a novel virus-host interaction in measles biology, it also has immediate applications for oncolytic virotherapy. It quickly became clear that this effect leads to rapid lysis of cancer cell lines *in vitro*. siRNA #2 can achieve near complete destruction of cancer cell monolayers at MOIs as low as 0.03, and far sooner than the control groups (Figure 11A). In cancer therapy, there is not only a desire for more potent therapeutics, but also a better safety profile. In the GM-38 fibroblast cell line used to represent healthy tissues, MeV Id-EGFP poorly fluoresces unlike in cancer cells (Figure 11B). Further, siRNA #2 does not sensitize the cells to greater MeV spread, despite being transfected efficiently as assessed by the Cy3-labelled siRNA control (data not shown). To quantify the extent of siRNA #2-mediated oncolysis, U-2 OS cells were infected at MOI 0.3 and cellular metabolic activity was measured with an XTT assay at 72 HPI (Figure 11C). In these types of assays, poor metabolic activity is a proxy for cell death, and it is clear siRNA #2 dramatically enhances MeV cytotoxicity. Thereafter, crystal violet staining was performed, and since most of the cells had lysed because of siRNA #2, there were far fewer adherent cells remaining (Figure 11D). Importantly, these experiments also show that siRNA #2 is not inherently cytotoxic in the absence of virus. As well, immunofluorescence staining for F-actin shows siRNA #2 does not affect cell morphology in uninfected U-2 OS cells (Figure 11E).

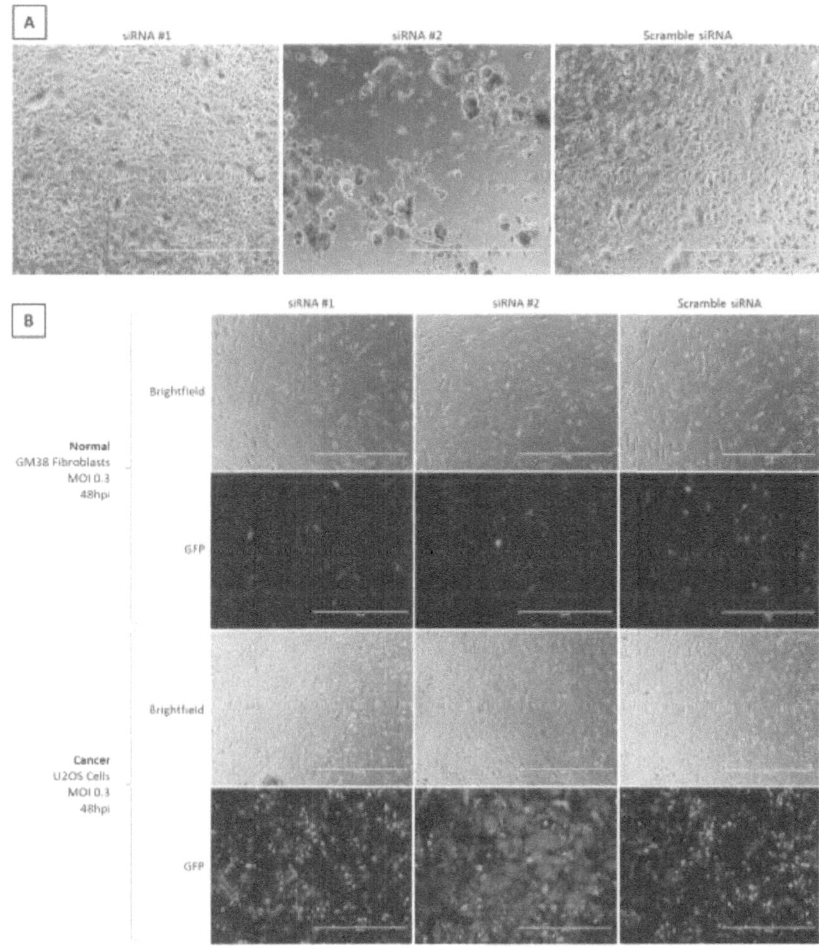

A
siRNA #1
siRNA #2
Scramble siRNA

B
siRNA #1
siRNA #2
Scramble siRNA
Brightfield
Normal
GM38 Fibroblasts
MOI 0.3
48hpi
GFP
Brightfield
Cancer
U2OS Cells
MOI 0.3
48hpi
GFP

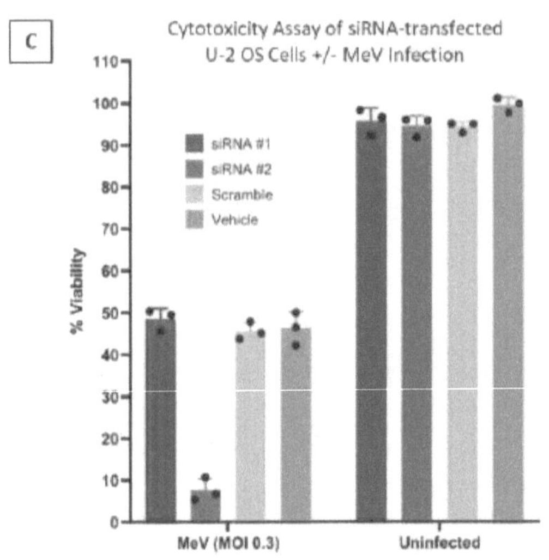

C
Cytotoxicity Assay of siRNA-transfected
U-2 OS Cells +/- MeV Infection
110
100
90
80
70
60
50
40
30
20
10
0
% Viability
siRNA #1
siRNA #2
Scramble
Vehicle
MeV (MOI 0.3)
Uninfected

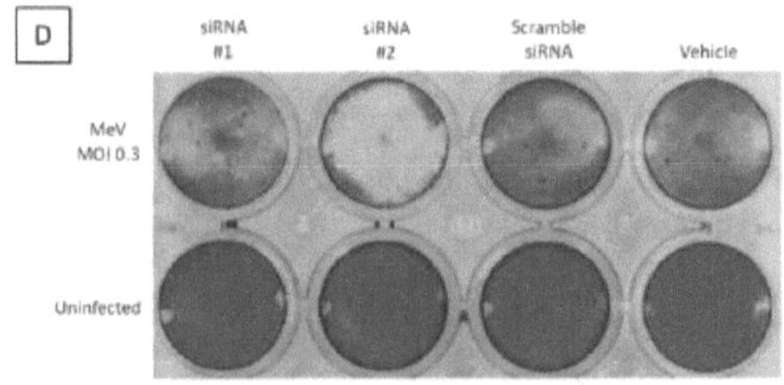

D
siRNA
#1
siRNA
#2
Scramble
siRNA
Vehicle
MeV
MOI 0.3
Uninfected

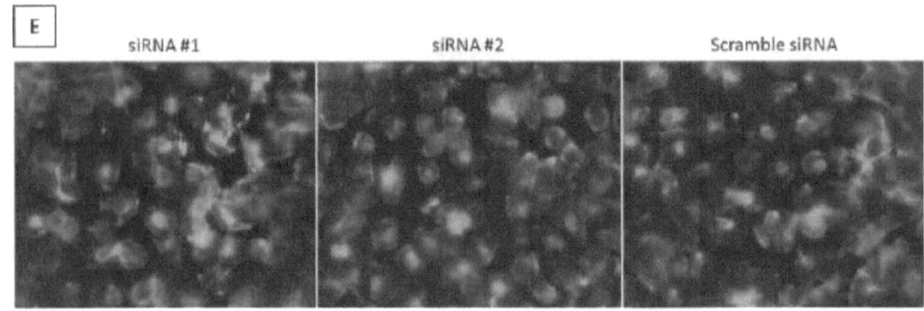

E
siRNA #1
siRNA #2
Scramble siRNA

Figure 11: siRNA #2-enhanced MeV spread boosts viral oncolysis *in vitro*. (A) PC-3 cells were infected with MeV (MOI 0.03) following siRNA transfection and brightfield images were captured at 72 HPI under a 4X objective. **(B)** Brightfield and GFP images of MeV Id-EGFP infection in a normal (GM-38) and cancerous (U-2 OS) cell line at 48 HPI following a six-hour siRNA transfection. Images were captured under a 4X objective. **(C)** XTT metabolic activity assay of infected and uninfected U-2 OS cells transfected with the siRNAs. Each data point represents the average of three replicates per condition. All samples were measured in triplicate. The data presented is representative of two independent experiments. **(D)** Crystal violet staining of cells infected with MeV (MOI 0.3) at 72 HPI after siRNA transfection. The plate shown is paired with the experiment in (C). **(E)** Phalloidin (F-actin) immunofluorescence staining of uninfected but siRNA-transfected U-2 OS cells to visualize cell morphology in the absence of virus. The image is merged with DAPI, thereby showing F-actin and nuclei. Images taken under 63X objective. Images are representative of two experiments in U-87 MG and U-2 OS cells.

10. siRNA #2 does not drastically enhance other OV platforms tested

There are several different viruses from diverse taxonomical groups currently being explored as cancer therapeutics, so siRNA #2 was screened with other available OV platforms from collaborators. Firstly, this was done to test whether the phenomenon caused by siRNA #2 could potentially benefit other virotherapeutics. Secondly, since phylogenetically dissimilar viruses have different host-pathogen interactions, finding viruses affected by siRNA #2 could provide insight into its underlying mechanisms.

Like MeV, VSV is a negative-sense single-stranded RNA virus in the mononegavirales order, and RIG-I is an important PRR in the host innate immune response to VSV infection.[121] However, knockdown of RIG-I with siRNAs yields only a small yet quantifiable increase in VSV-GFP signal area and intensity (Figures 12A, 12B, 12C). Both RIG-I siRNA #1 and #2 enhance VSV infection compared to controls, and siRNA #2 trends higher than siRNA #1 in PC-3 cells (Figures 12A, 12B), but the biological effect size and statistical significance is limited. A repetition experiment in U-2 OS cells showed no difference in VSV-GFP signal between siRNA #1 and #2 (Figure 12C). Therefore, firm conclusions cannot be drawn since the effect of siRNA #2 on VSV-GFP infection has been visually indistinguishable down the microscope, and there are inconsistencies across repetitions. This is in contract to MeV, where the effect size of enhanced spread caused by siRNA #2 is black-and-white.

Vaccinia virus (VacV) is a double-stranded DNA virus in the orthopoxvirus family. Being a DNA virus, RIG-I is not a key PRR in the host response to VacV infection, however RNA species produced in VacV-infected cells act as PAMPs recognized by RIG-I in a cell type-specific manner.[122] Only one cell line was tested for its RIG-I dependent inhibition of VacV, specifically PC-3 cells, because it was initially used as a model to study the siRNA #2-induced fusion phenotype. RIG-I silencing did not modulate VacV-GFP spread and fluorescence intensity, nor did siRNA #2 have any effect (Figure 12B). A confounding variable in this experiment is the extremely high MOI (clearly more than 0.01) that was inadvertently used, which likely did not provide any room for improvement. Further, this experiment should be repeated in A549 cells, where RIG-I is known to play a role in VacV infection.[122] Herpes simplex virus 1 (HSV-1) also has a double-stranded DNA genome, but RIG-I plays a larger role in its replication cycle.[123,124] With the exception of one positive result, siRNA #2 does not have a significant or reproducible effect on HSV-1 infection (Figure 12C).

Taken together, siRNA #2 has a clear benefit on MeV spread but does not significantly or consistently enhance the infection of three other OV platforms. This suggests the phenomenon caused by siRNA #2 impacts a process more specific to MeV. If this is true, it would be worthwhile screening siRNA #2 with other paramyxoviruses to see how phylogenetically stringent the effect is. It may also give valuable insight into the mechanism that is promoting MeV syncytial formation.

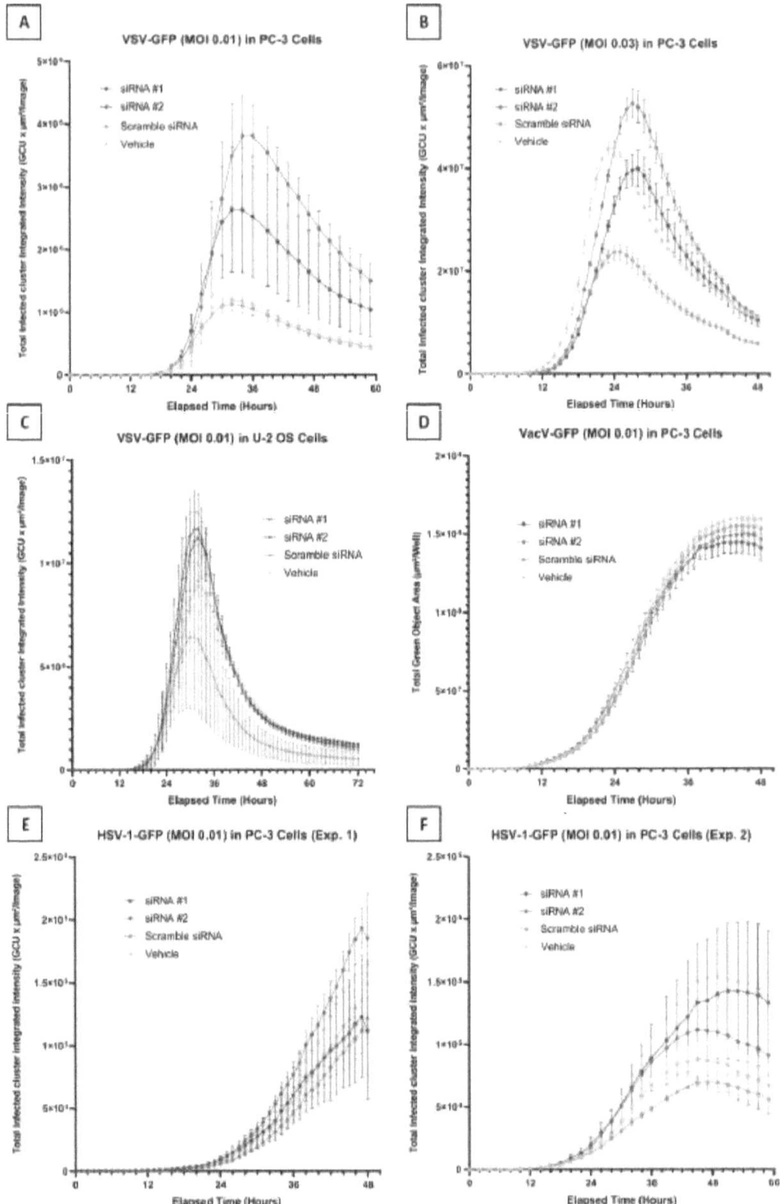

A
VSV-GFP (MOI 0.01) in PC-3 Cells
siRNA #1
siRNA #2
Scramble siRNA
Vehicle
Total infected cluster integrated intensity (GCU x µm²/Image)
Elapsed Time (Hours)

B
VSV-GFP (MOI 0.03) in PC-3 Cells
siRNA #1
siRNA #2
Scramble siRNA
Vehicle
Total infected cluster integrated intensity (GCU x µm²/Image)
Elapsed Time (Hours)

C
VSV-GFP (MOI 0.01) in U-2 OS Cells
siRNA #1
siRNA #2
Scramble siRNA
Vehicle
Total infected cluster integrated intensity (GCU x µm²/Image)
Elapsed Time (Hours)

D
VacV-GFP (MOI 0.01) in PC-3 Cells
siRNA #1
siRNA #2
Scramble siRNA
Vehicle
Total Green Object Area (µm²/Well)
Elapsed Time (Hours)

E
HSV-1-GFP (MOI 0.01) in PC-3 Cells (Exp. 1)
siRNA #1
siRNA #2
Scramble siRNA
Vehicle
Total infected cluster integrated intensity (GCU x µm²/Image)
Elapsed Time (Hours)

F
HSV-1-GFP (MOI 0.01) in PC-3 Cells (Exp. 2)
siRNA #1
siRNA #2
Scramble siRNA
Vehicle
Total infected cluster integrated intensity (GCU x µm²/Image)
Elapsed Time (Hours)

Figure 12: siRNA #2 does not significantly enhance VSV, VacV, or HSV-1 infection. **(A-C)** Three independent live cell imaging analysis (IncuCyte) plots of VSV-GFP infection following transfection with RIG-I siRNAs. Total GFP area of the well and signal intensity were measured and plotted against time. **(D)** GFP area of the well from VacV-GFP infection (MOI 0.01) following transfection with RIG-I siRNAs. Signal intensity was not included in the analysis; therefore, the metric solely quantifies viral spread over time. Repetition experiments were not performed. **(E-F)** Two independent experiments of HSV-1-GFP signal area and intensity after transfection with RIG-I siRNAs. In all live cell imaging experiments, each condition was performed in triplicate, and the data points are presented as the mean +/- SD.

Discussion

Clearly an siRNA has been identified with a peculiar effect on MeV infection. It has been characterized as enhancing MeV syncytia formation without increasing viral titers. The mechanism underlying this phenotype remains an enigma, but it does not directly involve the viral glycoproteins. It is suspected a host gene is suppressed through an siRNA-mediated sequence-dependent off-target effect which is then modulating MeV cell-cell fusion (Figure 13).

<u>Candidate Host Gene</u>   5′   NNNNNNNNNNNNCAACCGNNN 3′
<u>siRNA #2 Guide Strand</u>   3′ ttTCGGTTGGGATAATTCTGG   5′

<u>Seed Region</u>

Figure 13: Example of siRNA #2 guide-strand mediated off-target suppression of a host gene. The top sequence is a candidate host mRNA, which when knocked down, promotes enhanced MeV cell-cell fusion. The bottom sequence is the guide strand of siRNA #2, with the seed region highlighted. In this case there is perfect complementarity between the seed region and a small portion of the candidate host mRNA. Realistically, there might be non-canonical binding outside of the seed region that is still sufficient to facilitate suppression.

The effect caused by siRNA #2 on MeV infection seems quite unusual, yet, it is not the first time it has been reported. *Dietzel et al.* studied the effect of actin cytoskeleton dynamics on MeV maturation and showed actin cytoskeleton disruption leads to similar outcomes on MeV budding and cell-cell fusion as a result of impaired MeV matrix protein trafficking.[53] MeV matrix protein (M) is responsible for particle assembly and budding, which might relate to the reduction of virus particles detected in the supernatant following siRNA #2 transfection. MeV M also regulates glycoprotein fusion activity through its interaction with the cytoplasmic tails of H in the inner leaflet of the plasma membrane.[46]

This interaction inhibits cell-cell fusion so the glycoproteins can be incorporated into newly

forming particles. Thus, because the matrix protein bridges some of the information in

this book together, it may be involved in the spread phenotype. Future

experiments introducing MeV M into fusion assays along with F, H, and siRNA #2 will

be aimed at testing this hypothesis. Previous reports have shown that co-expression of

M decreases glycoprotein fusion activity in these assays, so if siRNA #2 is affecting M

somehow, then recovery of fusion activity would be seen by co-transfecting siRNA #2

with M, F, and H. An oversimplified model of this hypothesis is shown in Figure 14.

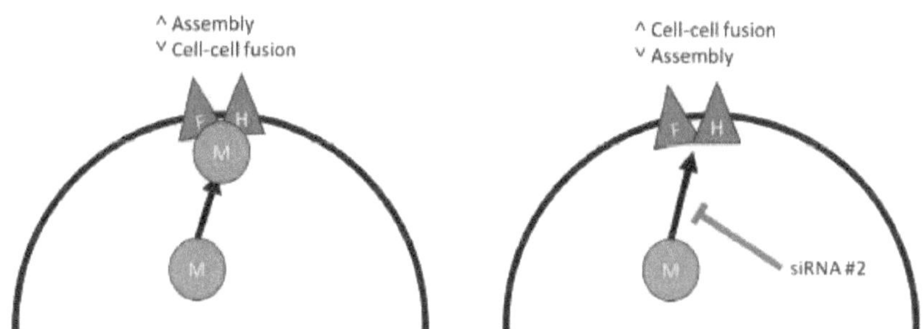

Figure 14: Oversimplified hypothesis of siRNA #2-mediated MeV M disruption. The white semicircles are cells, with the plasma membrane represented as the black outline. MeV F and H glycoproteins (coloured triangles) traffic to the plasma membrane where they cause cell-cell fusion between the infected cell and neighbouring cells. MeV M (coloured circle) traffics to the membrane by mechanisms not fully uncovered. When M associates with the cytoplasmic tails of F and H (as in the left diagram), viral assembly occurs and glycoprotein fusion activity is inhibited. The right diagram shows siRNA #2 acting on this process and its outcome. Interfering with M (as in the right diagram) is known to enhance cell-cell fusion and decrease viral assembly and budding.

Since siRNA #2 does not have meaningful sequence alignment with MeV M, or any other MeV gene for that matter, it would most likely interfere with a host gene that interacts with MeV M. If the host gene is involved in plasma membrane or nucleocytoplasmic trafficking of MeV M, there would be an observable subcellular redistribution of M which has not been seen in immunofluorescence experiments. It is quite possible MeV M is not involved in the phenotype. In this case, alternative experiments addressing MeV cell-cell fusion, maturation and egress should be considered. In line with this, one idea would be to quantify virus-like particle production in the presence of siRNA #2.

The conclusion that this siRNA is inducing off-target effects is rooted in the evidence that RIG-I knockdown is not sufficient for the enhanced fusion phenotype. With it only caused by one of three functional RIG-I siRNAs, as well as failure to block the siRNA #2-induced phenotype by overexpressing RIG-I, there is convincing evidence to support the notion of a sequence-dependent off-target effect. Recently, a paper was published which identified off-target effects from two *Trim58* shRNAs transduced into cells taken from *Trim58*[-/-] mice.[125] Since the off-target effects were induced by multiple non-overlapping shRNAs, plausible explanations are an shRNA-induced interferon response or saturation of endogenous RNAi machinery.[105,126] All experiments with siRNA #2 have been performed in RIG-I competent cell lines, but to be certain this is an off-target effect, the cell-cell fusion phenotype would need to be seen in RIG-I CRISPR-KO cells. Since a distinct phenotype is seen with only one of three non-overlapping siRNAs, it is likely to be caused by sequence-specific off-target effects. A549 RIG-I KO cells have been obtained courtesy of Dr. Marco Binder (German Cancer Research Center (DKFZ), Heidelberg,

Germany), and a RIG-I plasmid has been generated with three non-synonymous substitutions in the seed sequence of the siRNA target site (RIG-I^{mut}). With these mutations, RIG-I^{mut} will produce functional RIG-I protein but its mRNAs will be resistant to siRNA #2. If siRNA #2 definitively has off-target effects, the MeV spread phenotype would still occur in RIG-I$^{-/-}$ cells transiently expressing RIG-I^{mut}. These experiments are forthcoming, and should answer the off-target question. An alternative would be to use a cell line that is known to be RIG-I deficient. An established system used in RIG-I studies are the Huh7 and Huh7.5 cells.[93,127] Huh7.5 cells are RIG-I incompetent, so if siRNA #2 were to enhance syncytium formation in these cells it would almost certainly mean that this is mediated by off-target effects. These experiments would be dependent on whether the siRNA #2 fusion phenotype can be also be triggered in the isogenic Huh7 cell line.

Based on the results in this project, RIG-I knockdown does not lead to substantial improvements in MeV infection and is a weak target. Although MeV spread is strongly enhanced in A549 RIG KO cells, transient suppression using an siRNA in RIG-I competent cells only leads to a marginal increase in MeV replication, and this does not translate to a large effect on viral spread and cytotoxicity. This is consistent with a previous study, where knockdown with a RIG-I siRNA increased MeV replication by only 50% in H1299 and A549 cells.[128] Assuming RIG-I siRNA #2 is suppressing an off-target gene which then causes the enhanced spread phenotype, this other gene is a more promising target. The outcome of silencing this gene is enhanced MeV cell-cell fusion, which significantly improves viral oncolysis *in vitro*. If these cytotoxicity results can extrapolate from two-dimensional cell monolayers to three-dimensional tumours *in vivo*, this new finding could be utilized to improve MeV virotherapy. Several fusogenic oncolytic viruses form syncytia *in vivo* which is beneficial for therapeutic efficacy.[129]

Two options to incorporate the siRNA #2 sequence into MeV virotherapy are through engineering MeV-encoded amiRNAs as a monotherapy, or by delivering unmodified MeV virus in combination with siRNA #2-loaded nanoparticles. When extrapolating this work, the differences in target knockdown dynamics between siRNA transfection (prior to infection) and amiRNA expression from a replicating virus should be considered. This may only be an issue with targeting genes upstream in a signalling pathway, such as pattern recognition receptors (PRR), since the PRR is already present in the cell upon MeV entry. Saying that, it is logical to target downstream components of a signalling pathway, or a gene that is highly induced upon infection as part of a positive feedback loop. Achieving a by-stander effect, where amiRNAs are transported to neighbouring uninfected cells would be ideal for targeting early genes like PRRs. The cytoplasmic connections between cells called tunneling nanotubes (TNTs) might serve in such a by-stander effect. TNTs have once been studied with OVs, where they were shown to spread prodrug convertases through these channels.[130] Furthermore, endogenous microRNAs are known to traffic through TNTs,[131] so perhaps OV-encoded amiRNAs could also utilize TNTs to spread to naïve cells. This is now easier to study with recent methods that isolate TNT-mediated communication from other long- and short- range modes of intracytoplasmic delivery.[132]

Before developing the aforementioned therapeutic strategies, it is crucial to understand how siRNA #2 is promoting MeV syncytium formation. Elucidating the suspected off-target mRNA and mechanisms promoting syncytial formation may not only identify a novel virus-host interaction in MeV biology, but it could also open new avenues for future research into MeV biology. As well, since the phenotype induced by this siRNA appears to phenocopy some characteristics of MeV SSPE isolates, this research might shed light on the pathogenesis of this neurological disease.

Finding bystander host mRNAs suppressed by siRNA #2 will not be trivial because there are tens-of-thousands of RNAs expressed from the human genome. Usually off-target effects are found as false-positive hits in genome-wide siRNA screens and are rarely elucidated.[112,133] In one case, the off-target mRNA was found through the bioinformatics interface Genome-wide Enrichment of Seed Sequence matches (GESS).[133,134] However, inputting siRNA #2 guide and passenger strand sequences into the software was unproductive. Other siRNA off-target prediction tools exist but are either outdated or are not user-friendly.[135,136]

In one study, sequence-specific off-target shRNAs were transduced into cells that lack their respective targets followed by RNA sequencing.[137] Eleven targets were identified from cross-referencing alignment-based and read-based analytical methods, and most of these eleven targets were successfully validated by qPCR. The same alignment-based approach was used to compare the transcriptomes of samples transfected with siRNA #1 and #2, but what is informative about this study was the use of a secondary read-based analysis for cross-referencing to increase stringency. The read-based approach compares the abundance of specific reads between samples, and only the reads which differ substantially are subjected to an NCBI BLAST search to identify the gene it is derived from. Only genes that were commonly downregulated in both analyses were explored further, which lead to the identification of eleven off-target mRNAs, including ones that cause an off-target phenotype. This analytical approach should be replicated with the RNA sequencing data collected in this project.

The search for siRNA #2-mediated off-target mRNAs was focused on the primary criteria for siRNA off-target effects, which is perfect complementarity of the guide strand seed region with an off-target transcript. However, it could be that the passenger strand is mediating suppression too, and this plausibility should not be excluded.[112] Furthermore, seed-oriented prediction could miss non-canonical siRNA binding sites.[88] Most of the genes shown in Table 2 were identified from siRNA #2 sequence alignments using NCBI BLAST, but there are some exceptions. *ARPC5* was found from manually aligning the siRNA sequence with top hits in the RNA sequencing data. *FTL* and *ELMO1* were likewise found by aligning the siRNA sequence with 26 genes commonly downregulated more than two-fold in separate analyses. There could be other genes, like *ARPC5*, *FTL*, and *ELMO1* which have a perfect seed-match but are not found through NCBI BLAST. Essentially, this list of candidate genes in Table 2 is not exhaustive. Furthermore, the data is limited to the RNA level, when ideally the potential candidates should be assessed at the protein level. This is because siRNAs reduce target expression in at least two ways – through direct cleavage of the bound mRNA, or by stalling ribosome translation along the transcript.[138] With the former, off-target knockdown can be detected at the RNA level, but not if silencing is mediated through translational suppression. In either case, protein levels of the target are reduced so it would be best to use a proteomics approach.

The available RNA sequencing analysis is a useful tool to look at seed-matched candidates, but also other genes that might otherwise be missed. It is an invaluable resource, but so far it has only been analyzed manually. Deeper bioinformatics analysis can unveil potential pathways differentially regulated by siRNA #2, which could then be cross-referenced to the list of off-target gene candidates. Entering 750 genes with an expression foldchange greater than 1.5 into DAVID reveals a significant enrichment of ribosomal proteins, including those of the mitochondria, and genes involved in respiration. This could relate to the translational shutdown observed at 48 HPI in siRNA #2-transfected U-2 OS cells.

There is an apparent discrepancy in the two RPKM analyses, where *ARPC5* is an extreme example, and this is why the results of two independent analyses are shown in Table 2. It is also why a read-based analysis should be cross-referenced to increase stringency. Of the genes with a high fold change in expression (greater or less than two), only half are commonly shared between the two analyses. One factor could be that the reference databases are different, which makes the gene lists incongruent. When interpreting the data, it is more believable that the genes commonly sharing a high fold change in both analyses are biologically true. There are three genes with siRNA #2 seed complementarity that fit this category; *FTL, ELMO1*, and *MB*. Downregulation of *MB* was demonstrated by RT-PCR, and is currently the only gene where this has been reproducible. A western blot for MB would the next logical step to confirm siRNA #2-mediated MB suppression at the protein level, followed by transfection with a *MB*-specific siRNA to test whether *MB* suppression phenocopies siRNA #2. *FTL* and *ELMO1* have not been tested by RT-PCR, but it will be worthwhile considering their foldchange values are some of the largest in Table 2. As well, *FTL* is very highly expressed, with one of the highest RPKM values of all 19937 genes in the RNA sequencing datasets. Specifically, in mock-infected A549 cells, *FTL* is the single most highly expressed gene. A recent study ranked *FTL* as the third most highly expressed gene, accounting for 1.3% of total mRNAs.[139] Simply due to the extreme amount of *FTL* transcripts with high siRNA #2 sequence complementarity, stochastic passenger strand-mediated suppression events could be common. Also, three-fold downregulation of such a highly expressed gene might be more likely to have phenotypic consequences than a gene that is expressed at low levels.

With most of the differentially expressed candidates in Table 2, there is little to no literature supporting their involvement in viral infection. The primary function of Myoglobin is in oxygen storage for cardiac and muscle tissues, so it is unusual to see its expression outside of these cell types. *MB* has a perfect seed-match with the guide strand of siRNA #2, but the non-seed region is almost entirely composed of AU-rich mismatches. Mismatches towards the 3' end of the guide strand accelerate single-turnover cleavage rates, thereby enhancing target knockdown compared with complete complementarity.[80] Furthermore, a previous study of the nucleotide composition outside of the seed region showed AU mismatches are predictive of off-target annealing, which supports the likelihood that *MB* is suppressed as an siRNA #2 off-target effect.[79] *MB* has not been reported in virology, however hemoglobin (*HB*), which shares structural and functional similarities, has been reported to bind to the capsid protein of classical swine fever virus (CSFV).[140] HB depletion caused enhanced capsid protein expression, replication, and viral budding. Looking deeper into the mechanism of its antiviral activity, it was found HB activates IFN-β production and vice versa. Perhaps this relates to the increase in *MB* expression seen in MeV infection. HB was also shown to directly interact with RIG-I. Additionally, a recent study showed HB indeed has pleiotropic functions in innate immunity by promoting RIG-I activation.[141] Conversely, HB inhibits melanoma differentiation-associated protein 5 (MDA5), a pattern recognition receptor similar to RIG-I. *HB* overexpression negatively affects RNA viruses such as VSV, Sendai virus (SeV), and Newcastle disease virus (NDV).[141] SeV and NDV are taxonomically related to MeV, so *HB* might affect it as well. However, it would be farfetched extrapolating these studies to MeV and *MB*. Unfortunately, the SARS-CoV-2 pandemic interrupted the investigation into potential gene candidates. The only conclusion that can be drawn is that siRNA #2 appears to be suppressing *MB* at the RNA level, and though its relevance to the fusion phenotype is unknown and questionable, it is the first piece of evidence that siRNA #2 has off-target effects. The next two promising candidates based on the analyses in Table 2 are *FTL* and *ELMO1*.

ANXA8 is an intriguing candidate which has shown preliminary evidence of off-target suppression with siRNA #2, however a repetition experiment gave conflicting results. Though there are no reports of *ANXA8* in virology, the small body of research into this gene is relatively new, from which it has demonstrated pleiotropic effects. *ANXA8* is a member of the annexin family of Ca^{2+}-regulated membrane-binding proteins, with the ability to coordinate attachments between the membrane and actin cytoskeleton.[142] It is ectopically expressed in many human cancer cell lines, has oncogenic properties, and is a prognostic marker in some cancers.[143] What is most interesting is that *ANXA8* is closely related to other annexins which have important roles in MeV maturation and fusion. ANXA2 is currently the only known host factor to chaperone MeV M to the plasma membrane, which relates to the hypothesis that siRNA #2 is impairing a host factor involved in MeV egress.[52] *ANXA2* is also involved at different points of the life cycle of a wide range of human viruses.[144] Furthermore, ANXA1 directly interacts with MeV F and H and is necessary for efficient pore expansion during syncytium formation.[120] siRNA silencing of *ANXA1* consequently decreases MeV F-protein mediated syncytiogenesis. Lastly, one of the many functions of annexins is in plasma membrane repair and fusion. Considering *ANXA8* is a poorly characterized member of the annexin family, and the other annexins play a role in virology, including MeV, there is some rationale to hypothesize *ANXA8* dysregulation by siRNA #2 could lead to the enhanced fusion phenotype.

Studying the siRNA #2-induced phenotype may reveal new insight into MeV virus-host interactions, which would not only have implications for oncolytic virotherapy, but also in developing antiviral medicines. For the former, more work will be necessary to study this phenotype *in vivo*. It would be ideal to find the off-target gene before initiating animal experiments, where the phenotype could then be studied in a clean CRISPR-KO tumour model entirely lacking the gene. But if this is not possible, the siRNA sequence could be introduced into tumours *in vivo* through a variety of different methods. Firstly, as it relates to the original project, the siRNA sequence could be inserted into a MeV-encoded amiRNA which would be injected intratumorally. Alternatively, a cancer cell line could be stably transduced with an shRNA expressing the siRNA #2 sequence, then this cell line could be implanted to form tumours. The tumours would then be injected intratumorally with unmodified MeV and tumour volumes would be measured and compared to controls. Lastly, the siRNA could be transfected *in vivo* using a specialized reagent called Invivofectamine.[145–150] With both the MeV-amiRNA and Invivofectamine methods there will be incomplete penetrance of target knockdown in the tumour, though this would better emulate conditions in a therapeutic context. The cleaner experimental options are CRISPR-KO cells or stable shRNA cell lines because every cell in the tumour will be depleted of the target gene which will reduce confounding variables.

Enhancing cell-cell fusion should theoretically help MeV spread through the dense tumour microenvironment to ultimately debulk the lesion, however it remains to be seen how the tumour stroma (including the extracellular matrix) will impact its efficacy. All experiments so far have studied siRNA #2 in monocultures, but it might be relevant to evaluate its efficacy in a coculture system with stromal cells. As well, it is apparent some cancer cell lines are incredibly sensitive to the fusion phenotype whereas others are unaffected. Approximately twelve cancer cell lines have been tested with siRNA #2, and it would be interesting to expand this to a larger panel, like the NCI-60 panel, to identify other cell lines sensitive to this phenotype. Generally, it seemed the more susceptible a cell line is to MeV-induced cell-cell fusion, the greater the effect size from siRNA #2. This raises another important question - what are the cellular determinants for efficient MeV cell-cell fusion? It is certainly a multivariable phenomenon, including viral receptor (CD46) expression, virus replication and protein expression, as well as factors involved in MeV assembly and maturation. But for example, SW-620 cells are highly permissive to MeV infection, yet they do not readily form syncytia and are resistant to siRNA #2.[90] As well, Vero cells, which are from an African green monkey, are interferon defective and easily form syncytia, yet are refractory to siRNA #2. It is possible the off-target gene has weak sequence conservation between African green monkeys and its human homolog, thereby making the siRNA dysfunctional. Or it is possible this gene is not present in African green monkeys altogether. Without a better understanding of the predictors that predispose a cell's response to siRNA #2, there would be highly variable outcomes if this were to be developed as a therapeutic. Perhaps more research into the siRNA #2-induced phenotype will reveal factors that influence its efficacy. In the clinic, these predictive markers could be measured to determine whether the patient is likely to benefit from the therapy.

References

1.	Bianconi E, Piovesan A, Facchin F, et al. An estimation of the number of cells in the human body. *Ann Hum Biol*. 2013;40(6):463-471. doi:10.3109/03014460.2013.807878

2.	Canada PHA of, Canada S, Society CC, registries provincial/territorial cancer. Release notice - Canadian Cancer Statistics 2019 TT - Avis de publication - Statistiques canadiennes sur le cancer 2019. *Heal Promot chronic Dis Prev Canada Res policy Pract*. 2019;39(8-9):255. doi:10.24095/hpcdp.39.8/9.04

3.	Hanahan D, Weinberg RA. Hallmarks of cancer: the next generation. *Cell*. 2011;144(5):646-674. doi:10.1016/j.cell.2011.02.013

4.	Fisher R, Pusztai L, Swanton C. Cancer heterogeneity: implications for targeted therapeutics. *Br J Cancer*. 2013;108(3):479-485. doi:10.1038/bjc.2012.581

5.	Follain G, Herrmann D, Harlepp S, et al. Fluids and their mechanics in tumour transit: shaping metastasis. *Nat Rev Cancer*. 2020;20(2):107-124. doi:10.1038/s41568-019-0221-x

6.	Follain G, Osmani N, Azevedo AS, et al. Hemodynamic Forces Tune the Arrest, Adhesion, and Extravasation of Circulating Tumor Cells. *Dev Cell*. 2018;45(1):33-52.e12. doi:10.1016/j.devcel.2018.02.015

7.	Roth DB. V(D)J Recombination: Mechanism, Errors, and Fidelity. *Microbiol Spectr*. 2014;2(6). doi:10.1128/microbiolspec.MDNA3-0041-2014

8.	Lythe G, Callard RE, Hoare RL, Molina-París C. How many TCR clonotypes does a body maintain? *J Theor Biol*. 2016;389:214-224. doi:10.1016/j.jtbi.2015.10.016

9.	Klein L, Kyewski B, Allen PM, Hogquist KA. Positive and negative selection of the T cell repertoire: what thymocytes see (and don't see). *Nat Rev Immunol*. 2014;14(6):377-391. doi:10.1038/nri3667

10.	Maude SL, Teachey DT, Porter DL, Grupp SA. CD19-targeted chimeric antigen receptor T-cell therapy for acute lymphoblastic leukemia. *Blood*. 2015;125(26):4017-4023. doi:10.1182/blood-2014-12-580068

11.	Wei SC, Duffy CR, Allison JP. Fundamental Mechanisms of Immune Checkpoint Blockade Therapy. *Cancer Discov*. 2018;8(9):1069 LP - 1086. doi:10.1158/2159-8290.CD-18-0367

12.	Chang C-Y, Park H, Malone DC, et al. Immune Checkpoint Inhibitors and Immune-Related Adverse Events in Patients With Advanced Melanoma: A Systematic Review and Network Meta-analysis. *JAMA Netw Open*. 2020;3(3):e201611-e201611. doi:10.1001/jamanetworkopen.2020.1611

13.	Huang P-W, Chang JW-C. Immune checkpoint inhibitors win the 2018 Nobel Prize. *Biomed J*. 2019;42(5):299-306. doi:10.1016/j.bj.2019.09.002

14.	Chon HJ, Lee WS, Yang H, et al. Tumor Microenvironment Remodeling by Intratumoral Oncolytic Vaccinia Virus Enhances the Efficacy of Immune-Checkpoint Blockade. *Clin Cancer Res*. 2019;25(5):1612 LP - 1623. doi:10.1158/1078-0432.CCR-18-1932

15.	Engeland CE, Grossardt C, Veinalde R, et al. CTLA-4 and PD-L1 checkpoint blockade enhances oncolytic measles virus therapy. *Mol Ther*. 2014;22(11):1949-1959. doi:10.1038/mt.2014.160

16. Bourgeois-Daigneault M-C, Roy DG, Aitken AS, et al. Neoadjuvant oncolytic virotherapy before surgery sensitizes triple-negative breast cancer to immune checkpoint therapy. *Sci Transl Med*. 2018;10(422). http://stm.sciencemag.org/content/10/422/eaao1641.abstract.

17. Hardcastle J, Mills L, Malo CS, et al. Immunovirotherapy with measles virus strains in combination with anti-PD-1 antibody blockade enhances antitumor activity in glioblastoma treatment. *Neuro Oncol*. 2017;19(4):493-502. doi:10.1093/neuonc/now179

18. Stojdl DF, Lichty B, Knowles S, et al. Exploiting tumor-specific defects in the interferon pathway with a previously unknown oncolytic virus. *Nat Med*. 2000;6(7):821-825. doi:10.1038/77558

19. Stojdl DF, Lichty BD, tenOever BR, et al. VSV strains with defects in their ability to shutdown innate immunity are potent systemic anti-cancer agents. *Cancer Cell*. 2003;4(4):263-275. doi:https://doi.org/10.1016/S1535-6108(03)00241-1

20. McCart JA, Ward JM, Lee J, et al. Systemic Cancer Therapy with a Tumor-selective Vaccinia Virus Mutant Lacking Thymidine Kinase and Vaccinia Growth Factor Genes. *Cancer Res*. 2001;61(24):8751 LP - 8757. http://cancerres.aacrjournals.org/content/61/24/8751.abstract.

21. Bossow S, Grossardt C, Temme A, et al. Armed and targeted measles virus for chemovirotherapy of pancreatic cancer. *Cancer Gene Ther*. 2011;18(8):598-608. doi:10.1038/cgt.2011.30

22. Kelly E, Russell SJ. History of oncolytic viruses: genesis to genetic engineering. *Mol Ther*. 2007;15(4):651-659. doi:10.1038/sj.mt.6300108

23. Russell SJ, Peng KW. Measles virus for cancer therapy. *Curr Top Microbiol Immunol*. 2009;330:213-241. doi:10.1007/978-3-540-70617-5_11

24. Russell SJ, Babovic-Vuksanovic D, Bexon A, et al. Oncolytic Measles Virotherapy and Opposition to Measles Vaccination. *Mayo Clin Proc*. 2019;94(9):1834-1839. doi:10.1016/j.mayocp.2019.05.006

25. Roberts L. Why measles deaths are surging - and coronavirus could make it worse. *Nature*. 2020;580(7804):446-447. doi:10.1038/d41586-020-01011-6

26. Guerra FM, Bolotin S, Lim G, et al. The basic reproduction number (R(0)) of measles: a systematic review. *Lancet Infect Dis*. 2017;17(12):e420-e428. doi:10.1016/S1473-3099(17)30307-9

27. Zhao S, Lin Q, Ran J, et al. Preliminary estimation of the basic reproduction number of novel coronavirus (2019-nCoV) in China, from 2019 to 2020: A data-driven analysis in the early phase of the outbreak. *Int J Infect Dis IJID Off Publ Int Soc Infect Dis*. 2020;92:214-217. doi:10.1016/j.ijid.2020.01.050

28. Leung AK, Hon KL, Leong KF, Sergi CM. Measles: a disease often forgotten but not gone. *Hong Kong Med J = Xianggang yi xue za zhi*. 2018;24(5):512-520. doi:10.12809/hkmj187470

29. Laksono BM, de Vries RD, McQuaid S, Duprex WP, de Swart RL. Measles Virus Host Invasion and Pathogenesis. *Viruses*. 2016;8(8):210. doi:10.3390/v8080210

30. Garg RK, Mahadevan A, Malhotra HS, Rizvi I, Kumar N, Uniyal R. Subacute sclerosing panencephalitis. *Rev Med Virol*. 2019;29(5):e2058. doi:10.1002/rmv.2058

31. Benecke O, DeYoung SE. Anti-Vaccine Decision-Making and Measles Resurgence in the United States. *Glob Pediatr Heal*. 2019;6:2333794X19862949. doi:10.1177/2333794X19862949

32. Hussain A, Ali S, Ahmed M, Hussain S. The Anti-vaccination Movement: A Regression in Modern Medicine. *Cureus*. 2018;10(7):e2919. doi:10.7759/cureus.2919

33. ENDERS JF, PEEBLES TC. Propagation in tissue cultures of cytopathogenic agents from patients with measles. *Proc Soc Exp Biol Med Soc Exp Biol Med (New York, NY)*. 1954;86(2):277-286. doi:10.3181/00379727-86-21073

34. Tatsuo H, Ono N, Tanaka K, Yanagi Y SLAM (CDw150) is a cellular receptor for measles virus. *Nature*. 2000;406(6798):893-897. doi:10.1038/35022579

35. Noyce RS, Bondre DG, Ha MN, et al. Tumor cell marker PVRL4 (nectin 4) is an epithelial cell receptor for measles virus. *PLoS Pathog*. 2011;7(8):e1002240. doi:10.1371/journal.ppat.1002240

36. Nielsen L, Blixenkrone-Møller M, Thylstrup M, Hansen NJ, Bolt G. Adaptation of wild-type measles virus to CD46 receptor usage. *Arch Virol*. 2001;146(2):197-208. doi:10.1007/s007050170169

37. Cox RM, Plemper RK. Structure and organization of paramyxovirus particles. *Curr Opin Virol*. 2017;24:105-114. doi:10.1016/j.coviro.2017.05.004

38. Phan MVT, Schapendonk CME, Oude Munnink BB, Koopmans MPG, de Swart RL, Cotten M. Complete Genome Sequences of Six Measles Virus Strains. *Genome Announc*. 2018;6(13):e00184-18. doi:10.1128/genomeA.00184-18

39. Patterson JB, Thomas D, Lewicki H, Billeter MA, Oldstone MBA. V and C Proteins of Measles Virus Function as Virulence Factors in Vivo. *Virology*. 2000;267(1):80-89. doi:https://doi.org/10.1006/viro.1999.0118

40. Egelman EH, Wu SS, Amrein M, Portner A, Murti G. The Sendai virus nucleocapsid exists in at least four different helical states. *J Virol*. 1989;63(5):2233-2243. https://pubmed.ncbi.nlm.nih.gov/2539515.

41. Sauder CJ, Simonyan V, Ngo L, et al. Evidence that a polyhexameric genome length is preferred, but not strictly required, for efficient mumps virus replication. *Virology*. 2016;493:173-188. doi:10.1016/j.virol.2016.03.021

42. Matsumoto Y, Ohta K, Kolakofsky D, Nishio M. The control of paramyxovirus genome hexamer length and mRNA editing. *RNA*. 2018;24(4):461-467. doi:10.1261/rna.065243.117

43. Du Pont V, Jiang Y, Plemper RK. Bipartite interface of the measles virus phosphoprotein X domain with the large polymerase protein regulates viral polymerase dynamics. *PLOS Pathog*. 2019;15(8):e1007995. https://doi.org/10.1371/journal.ppat.1007995.

44. Aguilar HC, Henderson BA, Zamora JL, Johnston GP. Paramyxovirus Glycoproteins and the Membrane Fusion Process. *Curr Clin Microbiol reports*. 2016;3(3):142-154. doi:10.1007/s40588-016-0040-8

45.   Tahara M, Takeda M, Yanagi Y. Altered interaction of the matrix protein with the cytoplasmic tail of hemagglutinin modulates measles virus growth by affecting virus assembly and cell-cell fusion. *J Virol*. 2007;81(13):6827-6836. doi:10.1128/JVI.00248-07

46.   Wakimoto H, Shimodo M, Satoh Y, et al. F-actin modulates measles virus cell-cell fusion and assembly by altering the interaction between the matrix protein and the cytoplasmic tail of hemagglutinin. *J Virol*. 2013;87(4):1974-1984. doi:10.1128/JVI.02371-12

47.   Duan Z, Deng S, Ji X, Zhao J, Yuan C, Gao H. Nuclear localization of Newcastle disease virus matrix protein promotes virus replication by affecting viral RNA synthesis and transcription and inhibiting host cell transcription. *Vet Res*. 2019;50(1):22. doi:10.1186/s13567-019-0640-4

48.   Bankamp B, Fontana JM, Bellini WJ, Rota PA. Adaptation to cell culture induces functional differences in measles virus proteins. *Virol J*. 2008;5(1):129. doi:10.1186/1743-422X-5-129

49.   Cathomen T, Mrkic B, Spehner D, et al. A matrix-less measles virus is infectious and elicits extensive cell fusion: consequences for propagation in the brain. *EMBO J*. 1998;17(14):3899-3908. doi:10.1093/emboj/17.14.3899

50.   Runkler N, Pohl C, Schneider-Schaulies S, Klenk H-D, Maisner A. Measles virus nucleocapsid transport to the plasma membrane requires stable expression and surface accumulation of the viral matrix protein. *Cell Microbiol*. 2007;9(5):1203-1214. doi:10.1111/j.1462-5822.2006.00860.x

51.   Salditt A, Koethe S, Pohl C, et al. Measles virus M protein-driven particle production does not involve the endosomal sorting complex required for transport (ESCRT) system. *J Gen Virol*. 2010;91(Pt 6):1464-1472. doi:10.1099/vir.0.018523-0

52.   Koga R, Kubota M, Hashiguchi T, Yanagi Y, Ohno S. Annexin A2 Mediates the Localization of Measles Virus Matrix Protein at the Plasma Membrane. López S, ed. *J Virol*. 2018;92(10):e00181-18. doi:10.1128/JVI.00181-18

53.   Dietzel E, Kolesnikova L, Maisner A. Actin filaments disruption and stabilization affect measles virus maturation by different mechanisms. *Virol J*. 2013;10(1):249. doi:10.1186/1743-422X-10-249

54.   Grote D, Russell SJ, Cornu TI, et al. Live attenuated measles virus induces regression of human lymphoma xenografts in immunodeficient mice. *Blood*. 2001;97(12):3746-3754. doi:10.1182/blood.v97.12.3746

55.   Anderson BD, Nakamura T, Russell SJ, Peng K-W. High CD46 Receptor Density Determines Preferential Killing of Tumor Cells by Oncolytic Measles Virus. *Cancer Res*. 2004;64(14):4919 LP - 4926. doi:10.1158/0008-5472.CAN-04-0884

56.   Desjardins A, Gromeier M, Herndon JE, et al. Recurrent Glioblastoma Treated with Recombinant Poliovirus. *N Engl J Med*. 2018;379(2):150-161. doi:10.1056/NEJMoa1716435

57.   Russell SJ, Federspiel MJ, Peng K-W, et al. Remission of Disseminated Cancer After Systemic Oncolytic Virotherapy. *Mayo Clin Proc*. 2014;89(7):926-933. doi:10.1016/j.mayocp.2014.04.003

58.   Dispenzieri A, Tong C, LaPlant B, et al. Phase I trial of systemic administration of Edmonston strain of measles virus genetically engineered to express the sodium iodide

symporter in patients with recurrent or refractory multiple myeloma. *Leukemia.* 2017;31(12):2791-2798. doi:10.1038/leu.2017.120

59.   Galanis E, Hartmann LC, Cliby WA, et al. Phase I trial of intraperitoneal administration of an oncolytic measles virus strain engineered to express carcinoembryonic antigen for recurrent ovarian cancer. *Cancer Res.* 2010;70(3):875-882. doi:10.1158/0008-5472.CAN-09-2762

60.   Heinzerling L, Kunzi V, Oberholzer PA, Kundig T, Naim H, Dummer R. Oncolytic measles virus in cutaneous T-cell lymphomas mounts antitumor immune responses in vivo and targets interferon-resistant tumor cells. *Blood.* 2005;106(7):2287-2294. doi:10.1182/blood-2004-11-4558

61.   Msaouel P, Iankov ID, Allen C, et al. Noninvasive imaging and radiovirotherapy of prostate cancer using an oncolytic measles virus expressing the sodium iodide symporter. *Mol Ther.* 2009;17(12):2041-2048. doi:10.1038/mt.2009.218

62.   Penheiter AR, Wegman TR, Classic KL, et al. Sodium Iodide Symporter (NIS)-Mediated Radiovirotherapy for Pancreatic Cancer. *Am J Roentgenol.* 2010;195(2):341-349. doi:10.2214/AJR.09.3672

63.   Hutzen B, Pierson CR, Russell SJ, Galanis E, Raffel C, Studebaker AW. Treatment of medulloblastoma using an oncolytic measles virus encoding the thyroidal sodium iodide symporter shows enhanced efficacy with radioiodine. *BMC Cancer.* 2012;12:508. doi:10.1186/1471-2407-12-508

64.   Li H, Peng K-W, Russell SJ. Oncolytic measles virus encoding thyroidal sodium iodide symporter for squamous cell cancer of the head and neck radiovirotherapy. *Hum Gene Ther.* 2012;23(3):295-301. doi:10.1089/hum.2011.128

65.   Reddi H V, Madde P, McDonough SJ, et al. Preclinical efficacy of the oncolytic measles virus expressing the sodium iodide symporter in iodine non-avid anaplastic thyroid cancer: a novel therapeutic agent allowing noninvasive imaging and radioiodine therapy. *Cancer Gene Ther.* 2012;19(9):659-665. doi:10.1038/cgt.2012.47

66.   Ungerechts G, Springfeld C, Frenzke ME, et al. An immunocompetent murine model for oncolysis with an armed and targeted measles virus. *Mol Ther.* 2007;15(11):1991-1997. doi:10.1038/sj.mt.6300291

67.   Ungerechts G, Springfeld C, Frenzke ME, et al. Lymphoma chemovirotherapy: CD20-targeted and convertase-armed measles virus can synergize with fludarabine. *Cancer Res.* 2007;67(22):10939-10947. doi:10.1158/0008-5472.CAN-07-1252

68.   Ungerechts G, Frenzke ME, Yaiw K-C, Miest T, Johnston PB, Cattaneo R. Mantle cell lymphoma salvage regimen: synergy between a reprogrammed oncolytic virus and two chemotherapeutics. *Gene Ther.* 2010;17(12):1506-1516. doi:10.1038/gt.2010.103

69.   Lampe J, Bossow S, Weiland T, et al. An armed oncolytic measles vaccine virus eliminates human hepatoma cells independently of apoptosis. *Gene Ther.* 2013;20(11):1033-1041. doi:10.1038/gt.2013.28

70.   Kaufmann JK, Bossow S, Grossardt C, et al. Chemovirotherapy of Malignant Melanoma with a Targeted and Armed Oncolytic Measles Virus. *J Invest Dermatol.* 2013;133(4):1034-1042. doi:https://doi.org/10.1038/jid.2012.459

71.   Lange S, Lampe J, Bossow S, et al. A novel armed oncolytic measles vaccine virus for

the treatment of cholangiocarcinoma. *Hum Gene Ther*. 2013;24(5):554-564. doi:10.1089/hum.2012.136

72.   Maurer S, Salih HR, Smirnow I, Lauer UM, Berchtold S. Suicide genearmed measles vaccine virus for the treatment of AML. *Int J Oncol*. 2019;55(2):347-358. doi:10.3892/ijo.2019.4835

73.   Grote D, Cattaneo R, Fielding AK. Neutrophils contribute to the measles virus-induced antitumor effect: enhancement by granulocyte macrophage colony-stimulating factor expression. *Cancer Res*. 2003;63(19):6463-6468.

74.   Grossardt C, Engeland CE, Bossow S, et al. Granulocyte-Macrophage Colony-Stimulating Factor-Armed Oncolytic Measles Virus Is an Effective Therapeutic Cancer Vaccine. *Hum Gene Ther*. 2013;24(7):644-654. doi:10.1089/hum.2012.205

75.   Dietz L, Engeland CE. Immunomodulation in Oncolytic Measles Virotherapy BT - Oncolytic Viruses. In: Engeland CE, ed. New York, NY: Springer New York; 2020:111-126. doi:10.1007/978-1-4939-9794-7_7

76.   Speck T, Heidbuechel JPW, Veinalde R, et al. Targeted BiTE Expression by an Oncolytic Vector Augments Therapeutic Efficacy Against Solid Tumors. *Clin Cancer Res*. 2018;24(9):2128-2137. doi:10.1158/1078-0432.CCR-17-2651

77.   Veinalde R, Grossardt C, Hartmann L, et al. Oncolytic measles virus encoding interleukin-12 mediates potent antitumor effects through T cell activation. *Oncoimmunology*. 2017;6(4):e1285992. doi:10.1080/2162402X.2017.1285992

78.   Broughton JP, Lovci MT, Huang JL, Yeo GW, Pasquinelli AE. Pairing beyond the Seed Supports MicroRNA Targeting Specificity. *Mol Cell*. 2016;64(2):320-333. doi:10.1016/j.molcel.2016.09.004

79.   Kamola PJ, Nakano Y, Takahashi T, Wilson PA, Ui-Tei K. The siRNA Non-seed Region and Its Target Sequences Are Auxiliary Determinants of Off-Target Effects. *PLOS Comput Biol*. 2015;11(12):e1004656. https://doi.org/10.1371/journal.pcbi.1004656.

80.   Becker WR, Ober-Reynolds B, Jouravleva K, Jolly SM, Zamore PD, Greenleaf WJ. High-Throughput Analysis Reveals Rules for Target RNA Binding and Cleavage by AGO2. *Mol Cell*. 2019;75(4):741-755.e11. doi:10.1016/j.molcel.2019.06.012

81.   Freimer JW, Hu TJ, Blelloch R. Decoupling the impact of microRNAs on translational repression versus RNA degradation in embryonic stem cells. *Elife*. 2018;7. doi:10.7554/eLife.38014

82.   Bell JC, Kirn D. MicroRNAs fine-tune oncolytic viruses. *Nat Biotechnol*. 2008;26(12):1346-1348. doi:10.1038/nbt1208-1346

83.   Leber MF, Baertsch M-A, Anker SC, et al. Enhanced Control of Oncolytic Measles Virus Using MicroRNA Target Sites. *Mol Ther - Oncolytics*. 2018;9:30-40. doi:10.1016/j.omto.2018.04.002

84.   Loeb GB, Khan AA, Canner D, et al. Transcriptome-wide miR-155 binding map reveals widespread noncanonical microRNA targeting. *Mol Cell*. 2012;48(5):760-770. doi:10.1016/j.molcel.2012.10.002

85.   Eamens AL, McHale M, Waterhouse PM. The use of artificial microRNA technology to control gene expression in Arabidopsis thaliana. *Methods Mol Biol*. 2014;1062:211-224.

doi:10.1007/978-1-62703-580-4_11

86. Bhaskaran V, Yao Y, Bei F, Peruzzi P. Engineering, delivery, and biological validation of artificial microRNA clusters for gene therapy applications. *Nat Protoc*. 2019;14(12):3538-3553. doi:10.1038/s41596-019-0241-8

87. Jackson AL, Burchard J, Schelter J, et al. Widespread siRNA "off-target" transcript silencing mediated by seed region sequence complementarity. *RNA*. 2006;12(7):1179-1187. doi:10.1261/rna.25706

88. Seok H, Ham J, Jang E-S, Chi SW. MicroRNA Target Recognition: Insights from Transcriptome-Wide Non-Canonical Interactions. *Mol Cells*. 2016;39(5):375-381. doi:10.14348/molcells.2016.0013

89. Achard C, Boisgerault N, Delaunay T, et al. Sensitivity of human pleural mesothelioma to oncolytic measles virus depends on defects of the type I interferon response. *Oncotarget*. 2015;6(42):44892-44904. doi:10.18632/oncotarget.6285

90. Noll M, Berchtold S, Lampe J, Malek NP, Bitzer M, Lauer UM. Primary resistance phenomena to oncolytic measles vaccine viruses. *Int J Oncol*. 2013;43(1):103-112. doi:10.3892/ijo.2013.1914

91. Runge S, Sparrer KMJ, Lässig C, et al. In Vivo Ligands of MDA5 and RIG-I in Measles Virus-Infected Cells. *PLOS Pathog*. 2014;10(4):e1004081. https://doi.org/10.1371/journal.ppat.1004081.

92. Kolakofsky D, Kowalinski E, Cusack S. A structure-based model of RIG-I activation. *RNA*. 2012;18(12):2118-2127. doi:10.1261/rna.035949.112

93. Saito T, Hirai R, Loo Y-M, et al. Regulation of innate antiviral defenses through a shared repressor domain in RIG-I and LGP2. *Proc Natl Acad Sci U S A*. 2007;104(2):582-587. doi:10.1073/pnas.0606699104

94. Qi N, Shi Y, Zhang R, et al. Multiple truncated isoforms of MAVS prevent its spontaneous aggregation in antiviral innate immune signalling. *Nat Commun*. 2017;8(1):15676. doi:10.1038/ncomms15676

95. Soye KJ, Trottier C, Richardson CD, Ward BJ, Miller WH. RIG-I Is Required for the Inhibition of Measles Virus by Retinoids. Albert ML, ed. *PLoS One*. 2011;6(7):e22323. doi:10.1371/journal.pone.0022323

96. Kelly JT, Human S, Alderman J, et al. BST2/Tetherin Overexpression Modulates Morbillivirus Glycoprotein Production to Inhibit Cell-Cell Fusion. *Viruses*. 2019;11(8). doi:10.3390/v11080692

97. Kakihara Y, Houry WA. The R2TP complex: discovery and functions. *Biochim Biophys Acta*. 2012;1823(1):101-107. doi:10.1016/j.bbamcr.2011.08.016

98. Katoh H, Sekizuka T, Nakatsu Y, et al. The R2TP complex regulates paramyxovirus RNA synthesis. *PLoS Pathog*. 2019;15(5):e1007749. doi:10.1371/journal.ppat.1007749

99. Carmichael JC, Yokota H, Craven RC, Schmitt A, Wills JW. The HSV-1 mechanisms of cell-to-cell spread and fusion are critically dependent on host PTP1B. *PLoS Pathog*. 2018;14(5):e1007054. doi:10.1371/journal.ppat.1007054

100. Nguyên TL-A, Abdelbary H, Arguello M, et al. Chemical targeting of the innate antiviral

response by histone deacetylase inhibitors renders refractory cancers sensitive to viral oncolysis. *Proc Natl Acad Sci U S A*. 2008;105(39):14981-14986. doi:10.1073/pnas.0803988105

101. Veitia RA. Exploring the molecular etiology of dominant-negative mutations. *Plant Cell*. 2007;19(12):3843-3851. doi:10.1105/tpc.107.055053

102. Gack MU, Kirchhofer A, Shin YC, et al. Roles of RIG-I N-terminal tandem CARD and splice variant in TRIM25-mediated antiviral signal transduction. *Proc Natl Acad Sci U S A*. 2008;105(43):16743-16748. doi:10.1073/pnas.0804947105

103. Hu J, Nistal-Villán E, Voho A, et al. A common polymorphism in the caspase recruitment domain of RIG-I modifies the innate immune response of human dendritic cells. *J Immunol*. 2010;185(1):424-432. doi:10.4049/jimmunol.0903291

104. Caffrey DR, Zhao J, Song Z, et al. siRNA Off-Target Effects Can Be Reduced at Concentrations That Match Their Individual Potency. *PLoS One*. 2011;6(7):e21503. https://doi.org/10.1371/journal.pone.0021503.

105. Khan AA, Betel D, Miller ML, Sander C, Leslie CS, Marks DS. Transfection of small RNAs globally perturbs gene regulation by endogenous microRNAs. *Nat Biotechnol*. 2009;27(6):549-555. doi:10.1038/nbt.1543

106. Inoue Y, Sato H, Fujita K, Tsukiyama-Kohara K, Yoneda M, Kai C. Selective translation of the measles virus nucleocapsid mRNA by la protein. *Front Microbiol*. 2011;2:173. doi:10.3389/fmicb.2011.00173

107. Singh BK, Li N, Mark AC, Mateo M, Cattaneo R, Sinn PL. Cell-to-Cell Contact and Nectin-4 Govern Spread of Measles Virus from Primary Human Myeloid Cells to Primary Human Airway Epithelial Cells. Lyles DS, ed. *J Virol*. 2016;90(15):6808 LP - 6817. doi:10.1128/JVI.00266-16

108. Naim HY, Ehler E, Billeter MA. Measles virus matrix protein specifies apical virus release and glycoprotein sorting in epithelial cells. *EMBO J*. 2000;19(14):3576-3585. doi:10.1093/emboj/19.14.3576

109. Yu X, Shahriari S, Li H-M, Ghildyal R. Measles Virus Matrix Protein Inhibits Host Cell Transcription. *PLoS One*. 2016;11(8):e0161360-e0161360. doi:10.1371/journal.pone.0161360

110. Hasegawa Y, Mao W, Saha S, et al. Luciferase shRNA Presents off-Target Effects on Voltage-Gated Ion Channels in Mouse Hippocampal Pyramidal Neurons. *eneuro*. 2017;4(5):ENEURO.0186-17.2017. doi:10.1523/ENEURO.0186-17.2017

111. Tschuch C, Schulz A, Pscherer A, et al. Off-target effects of siRNA specific for GFP. *BMC Mol Biol*. 2008;9:60. doi:10.1186/1471-2199-9-60

112. Schultz N, Marenstein DR, De Angelis DA, et al. Off-target effects dominate a large-scale RNAi screen for modulators of the TGF-β pathway and reveal microRNA regulation of TGFBR2. *Silence*. 2011;2:3. doi:10.1186/1758-907X-2-3

113. Gournier H, Goley ED, Niederstrasser H, Trinh T, Welch MD. Reconstitution of human Arp2/3 complex reveals critical roles of individual subunits in complex structure and activity. *Mol Cell*. 2001;8(5):1041-1052. doi:10.1016/s1097-2765(01)00393-8

114. Kristiansen G, Hu J, Wichmann D, et al. Endogenous Myoglobin in Breast Cancer Is

Hypoxia-inducible by Alternative Transcription and Functions to Impair Mitochondrial Activity: A ROLE IN TUMOR SUPPRESSION? . *J Biol Chem* . 2011;286(50):43417-43428. doi:10.1074/jbc.M111.227553

115. Bicker A, Brahmer AM, Meller S, Kristiansen G, Gorr TA, Hankeln T. The Distinct Gene Regulatory Network of Myoglobin in Prostate and Breast Cancer. *PLoS One.* 2015;10(11):e0142662-e0142662. doi:10.1371/journal.pone.0142662

116. Huttlin EL, Ting L, Bruckner RJ, et al. The BioPlex Network: A Systematic Exploration of the Human Interactome. *Cell.* 2015;162(2):425-440. doi:10.1016/j.cell.2015.06.043

117. Summer S, Smirnova A, Gabriele A, et al. YBEY is an essential biogenesis factor for mitochondrial ribosomes. *Nucleic Acids Res.* March 2020. doi:10.1093/nar/gkaa148

118. Huang DW, Sherman BT, Lempicki RA. Bioinformatics enrichment tools: paths toward the comprehensive functional analysis of large gene lists. *Nucleic Acids Res.* 2009;37(1):1-13. doi:10.1093/nar/gkn923

119. Huang DW, Sherman BT, Lempicki RA. Systematic and integrative analysis of large gene lists using DAVID bioinformatics resources. *Nat Protoc.* 2009;4(1):44-57. doi:10.1038/nprot.2008.211

120. Ciechonska M, Key T, Duncan R. Efficient reovirus- and measles virus-mediated pore expansion during syncytium formation is dependent on annexin A1 and intracellular calcium. *J Virol.* 2014;88(11):6137-6147. doi:10.1128/JVI.00121-14

121. Gack MU, Nistal-Villán E, Inn K-S, García-Sastre A, Jung JU. Phosphorylation-Mediated Negative Regulation of RIG-I Antiviral Activity. *J Virol.* 2010;84(7):3220 LP - 3229. doi:10.1128/JVI.02241-09

122. Myskiw C, Arsenio J, Booy EP, et al. RNA species generated in vaccinia virus infected cells activate cell type-specific MDA5 or RIG-I dependent interferon gene transcription and PKR dependent apoptosis. *Virology.* 2011;413(2):183-193. doi:https://doi.org/10.1016/j.virol.2011.01.034

123. Liu Y, Goulet M-L, Sze A, et al. RIG-I-Mediated STING Upregulation Restricts Herpes Simplex Virus 1 Infection. *J Virol.* 2016;90(20):9406-9419. doi:10.1128/JVI.00748-16

124. Crill EK, Furr-Rogers SR, Marriott I. RIG-I is required for VSV-induced cytokine production by murine glia and acts in combination with DAI to initiate responses to HSV-1. *Glia.* 2015;63(12):2168-2180. doi:10.1002/glia.22883

125. Traxler EA, Thom CS, Yao Y, Paralkar V, Weiss MJ. Nonspecific inhibition of erythropoiesis by short hairpin RNAs. *Blood.* 2018;131(24):2733-2736. doi:10.1182/blood-2018-03-841304

126. Machitani M, Sakurai F, Wakabayashi K, Takayama K, Tachibana M, Mizuguchi H. Type I Interferons Impede Short Hairpin RNA-Mediated RNAi via Inhibition of Dicer-Mediated Processing to Small Interfering RNA. *Mol Ther Nucleic Acids.* 2017;6:173-182. doi:10.1016/j.omtn.2016.12.007

127. Sumpter Jr R, Loo Y-M, Foy E, et al. Regulating intracellular antiviral defense and permissiveness to hepatitis C virus RNA replication through a cellular RNA helicase, RIG-I. *J Virol.* 2005;79(5):2689-2699. doi:10.1128/JVI.79.5.2689-2699.2005

128. Xia M, Gonzalez P, Li C, et al. Mitophagy Enhances Oncolytic Measles Virus Replication

by Mitigating DDX58/RIG-I-Like Receptor Signaling. Lyles DS, ed. *J Virol*. 2014;88(9):5152-5164. doi:10.1128/JVI.03851-13

129. Burton C, Bartee E. Syncytia Formation in Oncolytic Virotherapy. *Mol Ther - Oncolytics*. 2019;15:131-139. doi:https://doi.org/10.1016/j.omto.2019.09.006

130. Ady J, Thayanithy V, Mojica K, et al. Tunneling nanotubes: an alternate route for propagation of the bystander effect following oncolytic viral infection. *Mol Ther oncolytics*. 2016;3:16029. doi:10.1038/mto.2016.29

131. Lu JJ, Yang WM, Li F, Zhu W, Chen Z. Tunneling Nanotubes Mediated microRNA-155 Intercellular Transportation Promotes Bladder Cancer Cells' Invasive and Proliferative Capacity. *Int J Nanomedicine*. 2019;14:9731-9743. doi:10.2147/IJN.S217277

132. Thayanithy V, O'Hare P, Wong P, et al. A transwell assay that excludes exosomes for assessment of tunneling nanotube-mediated intercellular communication. *Cell Commun Signal*. 2017;15(1):46. doi:10.1186/s12964-017-0201-2

133. Adamson B, Smogorzewska A, Sigoillot FD, King RW, Elledge SJ. A genome-wide homologous recombination screen identifies the RNA-binding protein RBMX as a component of the DNA-damage response. *Nat Cell Biol*. 2012;14(3):318-328. doi:10.1038/ncb2426

134. Yilmazel B, Hu Y, Sigoillot F, et al. Online GESS: prediction of miRNA-like off-target effects in large-scale RNAi screen data by seed region analysis. *BMC Bioinformatics*. 2014;15:192. doi:10.1186/1471-2105-15-192

135. Zhao W, Lane T. SiRNA Off-Target Search: A Hybrid q-Gram Based Filtering Approach. In: *Proceedings of the 5th International Workshop on Bioinformatics*. BIOKDD '05. New York, NY, USA: Association for Computing Machinery; 2005:54–60. doi:10.1145/1134030.1134040

136. Lück S, Kreszies T, Strickert M, Schweizer P, Kuhlmann M, Douchkov D. siRNA-Finder (si-Fi) Software for RNAi-Target Design and Off-Target Prediction . *Front Plant Sci* . 2019;10:1023. https://www.frontiersin.org/article/10.3389/fpls.2019.01023.

137. Putzbach W, Gao QQ, Patel M, et al. Many si/shRNAs can kill cancer cells by targeting multiple survival genes through an off-target mechanism. *Elife*. 2017;6. doi:10.7554/eLife.29702

138. Valencia-Sanchez MA, Liu J, Hannon GJ, Parker R. Control of translation and mRNA degradation by miRNAs and siRNAs. *Genes Dev*. 2006;20(5):515-524. doi:10.1101/gad.1399806

139. Zhao S, Ye Z, Stanton R. Misuse of RPKM or TPM normalization when comparing across samples and sequencing protocols. *RNA*. 2020;26(8):903-909. doi:10.1261/rna.074922.120

140. Li D, Dong H, Li S, et al. Hemoglobin subunit beta interacts with the capsid protein and antagonizes the growth of classical swine fever virus. *J Virol*. 2013;87(10):5707-5717. doi:10.1128/JVI.03130-12

141. Yang Q, Bai S-Y, Li L-F, et al. Human Hemoglobin Subunit Beta Functions as a Pleiotropic Regulator of RIG-I/MDA5-Mediated Antiviral Innate Immune Responses. Williams BRG, ed. *J Virol*. 2019;93(16):e00718-19. doi:10.1128/JVI.00718-19

142. Rentero C, Blanco-Muñoz P, Meneses-Salas E, Grewal T, Enrich C. Annexins-Coordinators of Cholesterol Homeostasis in Endocytic Pathways. *Int J Mol Sci*. 2018;19(5):1444. doi:10.3390/ijms19051444

143. Hata H, Tatemichi M, Nakadate T. Involvement of annexin A8 in the properties of pancreatic cancer. *Mol Carcinog*. 2014;53(3):181-191. doi:10.1002/mc.21961

144. Taylor JR, Skeate JG, Kast WM. Annexin A2 in Virus Infection . *Front Microbiol* . 2018;9:2954. https://www.frontiersin.org/article/10.3389/fmicb.2018.02954.

145. Chen R-Y, Chen H-X, Lin J-X, et al. In-vivo transfection of pcDNA3.1-IGFBP7 inhibits melanoma growth in mice through apoptosis induction and VEGF downexpression. *J Exp Clin Cancer Res*. 2010;29(1):13. doi:10.1186/1756-9966-29-13

146. Khan S, Ebeling MC, Zaman MS, et al. MicroRNA-145 targets MUC13 and suppresses growth and invasion of pancreatic cancer. *Oncotarget*. 2014;5(17):7599-7609. doi:10.18632/oncotarget.2281

147. Bartolomé-Izquierdo N, de Yébenes VG, Álvarez-Prado AF, et al. miR-28 regulates the germinal center reaction and blocks tumor growth in preclinical models of non-Hodgkin lymphoma. *Blood*. 2017;129(17):2408-2419. doi:10.1182/blood-2016-08-731166

148. Vidal SJ, Rodriguez-Bravo V, Quinn SA, et al. A targetable GATA2-IGF2 axis confers aggressiveness in lethal prostate cancer. *Cancer Cell*. 2015;27(2):223-239. doi:10.1016/j.ccell.2014.11.013

149. Chen R-Y, Chen H-X, Jian P, et al. Intratumoral injection of pEGFC1-IGFBP7 inhibits malignant melanoma growth in C57BL/6J mice by inducing apoptosis and down-regulating VEGF expression. *Oncol Rep*. 2010;23(4):981-988. doi:10.3892/or_00000723

150. Kim CJ, Terado T, Tambe Y, et al. Anti-oncogenic activities of cyclin D1b siRNA on human bladder cancer cells via induction of apoptosis and suppression of cancer cell stemness and invasiveness. *Int J Oncol*. 2018;52(1):231-240. doi:10.3892/ijo.2017.4194

Contributions of Collaborators

Stefanie Prien, research technician in the laboratory of Dr. Guy Ungerechts (National Center for Tumour Diseases Heidelberg, Heidelberg, Germany) received, cultured, and infected A549 RIG-I$^{-/-}$ KO cells with MeV-GFP and collected fluorescent microscopy images that contributed to Figure 1C.

Vickey Gilchrist, Master's student in the laboratory of Dr. Tommy Alain (Children's Hospital of Eastern Ontario Research Institute, Ottawa, Canada) built the GFP mask shown in Figure 1H that allowed for accurate quantification of fluorescent signal from GFP-tagged measles virus infection of PC-3 cells using IncuCyte Live Cell Imaging Analysis.

Adrian Pelin, PhD student in the laboratory of Dr. John Bell (Ottawa Hospital Research Institute, Ottawa, Canada) submitted the prepared RNA samples for RNA sequencing and analyzed the raw data to form a list of RPKM values that contributed to Table 2A.

Huy-Dung Hoang, PhD student in the laboratory of Dr. Tommy Alain (Children's Hospital of Eastern Ontario Research Institute, Ottawa, Canada) independently analyzed the RNA sequencing raw data to form a list of RPKM values that contributed to Table 2B.

Dr. Tommy Alain, Associate Professor and Scientist (Children's Hospital of Eastern Ontario Research Institute, Ottawa, Canada) performed the ^{35}S radioisotope labelling experiment on siRNA-transfected and MeV-infected samples shown in Figure 7B.

Dr. Tyson Graber, Research Associate in the laboratory of Dr. Tommy Alain (Children's Hospital of Eastern Ontario Research Institute, Ottawa, Canada) imaged the fixed immunofluorescence microscopy slides with a confocal microscope which contributed to Figure 8.

Russell John Robert Barkley

PhD Candidate, Biomedical and Biological Sciences – Cornell University

EDUCATION

Doctor of Philosophy (PhD) in Biomedical and Biological Sciences   2020 – Present
Specializing in Immunology and Infectious Disease
Cornell University | Ithaca, New York, United States of America

Master of Science (MSc) in Microbiology and Immunology   2018 – 2020
Investigation of an Oncolytic MeV Cell-Cell Fusion Phenomenon Induced by an siRNA
University of Ottawa | Ottawa, Canada
book Supervisor: Dr. Guy Ungerechts – Clinician Scientist, NCT Heidelberg

Honours Bachelor of Science (BSc) in Biomedical Science (CO-OP)   2013 - 2018
summa cum laude
University of Ottawa | Ottawa, Canada
book Supervisor: Dr. John C. Bell – Senior Scientist, OHRI

PUBLICATIONS, RESEARCH & PRESENTATIONS

PUBLICATIONS

Leber MF, Baertsch MA, Anker S, Henkel L, Singh H, Bossow S, Engeland C, **Barkley R**, Hoyler B, Albert J, Springfield C, Jäger D, Von Kalle C, Ungerechts G. Enhanced Control of Oncolytic Measles Virus Using MicroRNA Target Sites. *Molecular Therapy Oncolytics*. 2018 Jun 29; 9: 30-40. 30-40. Epub 2018 Apr 12. doi: 10.1016/j.omto.2018.04.002. PMCID: PMC6026446

Leber MF, Neault S, Jirovec E, **Barkley R**, Said A, Bell JC, Ungerechts G. Engineering and combining oncolytic measles virus for cancer therapy. *Cytokine & Growth Factor Reviews*. Epub 2020 July 3. doi: 10.1016/j.cytogfr.2020.07.005. PMCID: PMC7333629

LABORATORY EXPERIENCE

Graduate Student   September 2018 – August 2020
OHRI Centre for Innovative Cancer Therapeutics | Ottawa, Ontario
Supervisor: Dr. Guy Ungerechts

Volunteer Research Student   September 2018 – August 2020
Children's Hospital of Eastern Ontario Research Institute | Ottawa, Ontario
Supervisor: Dr. Tommy Alain

CO-OP Student   **May 2017 – December 2017**
National Center for Tumour Diseases | Heidelberg, Germany
Supervisor: Prof. Dr. Dr. Guy Ungerechts

CO-OP Student   **January 2016 – September 2016**
OHRI Centre for Innovative Cancer Therapeutics | Ottawa, Ontario
Supervisor: Dr. John Bell

Undergraduate Research Opportunity Student   **August 2015 – March 2016**
Hearing Research Laboratory, University of Ottawa | Ottawa, Ontario
Supervisor: Dr. Amineh Koravand

ORAL PRESENTATIONS

Work in Progress (WIP) Seminar – OHRI Centre for Innovative Cancer Therapeutics, 9 April 2020, Ottawa ON. Online seminar.

Work in Progress (WIP) Seminar – OHRI Centre for Innovative Cancer Therapeutics, 6 June 2019, Ottawa ON.

Work in Progress (WIP) Seminar – CHEO Research Institute, 6 February 2019, Ottawa ON.

Molecular Journal Club – OHRI Centre for Innovative Cancer Therapeutics, 7 November 2018, Ottawa ON.

CO-OP Presentation – National Center for Tumour Diseases, 14 December 2017, Heidelberg, Germany.

CO-OP Presentation – National Center for Tumour Diseases (NCT), 21 June 2017, Heidelberg, Germany.

Bridging Academic Minds: Science in 2025 Speaker Series – Undergraduate Science Case Competition, 24-26 March 2017, London, Ontario.

CO-OP Presentation – OHRI Centre for Innovative Cancer Therapeutics, 5 August 2016, Ottawa, ON.

CO-OP Presentation – OHRI Centre for Innovative Cancer Therapeutics, 17 June 2016, Ottawa, ON.

POSTER PRESENTATIONS

Barkley R, Leber MF, Prien S, Neault S, Gilchrist V, Bell JC, Alain T (2019). Ungerechts G, Boosting Measles Virus Oncolysis through RNAi, OHRI Research Day 2019, November 7 2019, Ottawa, ON.

Barkley R, Leber MF, Prien S, Neault S, Gilchrist V, Bell JC, Alain T, Ungerechts G, Boosting Measles Virus Oncolysis through RNAi, Canadian Cancer Research Conference 2019, 3-5 November 2019, Ottawa, ON.

Barkley R, Leber MF, Prien S, Neault S, Gilchrist V, Bell JC, Alain T, Ungerechts G, Boosting Measles Virus Oncolysis through RNAi, Summit for Cancer Immunotherapy, 20-23 October 2019, Victoria, BC.

Barkley R,_Leber MF, Neault S, Bell JC, Alain T, Ungerechts G, Arming Oncolytic Measles Virus with Therapeutic Artificial MicroRNAs, University of Ottawa, BMI Poster Day, 2 May 2019, Ottawa, ON.

Barkley R, Keller, BA, Pelin, A, Wang, J, LeBoeuf, F, Nessim, C, Ilkow, C, Atkins, HA, Bell, JC, Optimizing the Oncolytic Vaccinia Virus Backbone, and Characterizing Plaque Size Phenotypes Caused by Single Gene Knockouts, Honours book Poster Presentation, 29 April 2017, Ottawa, ON.

Barkley R, Laight B, Jirovec A, Banville A, Recombinant Wolbachia Reduces ZIKA Replication and Dissemination via Inflammasome Inhibition, University of Western Ontario, Undergraduate Science Case Competition, 24-26 March 2017, London, Ontario.

Keller, BA, **Barkley R**, Pelin, A, Wang, J, LeBoeuf, F, Nessim, C, Ilkow, C, Atkins, HA, Bell, JC, Optimizing the Vaccinia backbone for use as an oncolytic virus using insertional mutagenesis, Terry Fox Research Institute, Ontario Node Symposium, 5 Dec 2016, Toronto, ON.

Keller, BA, Pelin, A, **Barkley R**, Budhram B, Wang, J, Le Boeuf, F, Nessim C, Ilkow C, Atkins HA, Bell, JC, Random mutagenesis of Vaccinia virus uncovers novel clinical candidate oncolytic backbones with unique phenotypes, OHRI Research Day 2016, 10 Nov 2016, Ottawa, ON.

Keller, BA, Pelin, A, **Barkley R**, Budhram B, Wang, J, Le Boeuf, F, Nessim C, Ilkow C, Atkins HA, Bell, JC, Augmenting the anti-tumour immunogenicity of Vaccinia virus using transposon-mediated mutagenesis, Summit for Cancer Immunotherapy, 26-29 June 2016, Halifax, Nova Scotia.

Keller, BA, Pelin, A, **Barkley R**, Wang, J, Le Boeuf, F, Nessim C, Ilkow C, Atkins HA, Bell, JC, Creating and characterizing a transposon-mutagenized library of Vaccinia virus clones for the treatment of human cancer, Terry Fox Research Institute Annual Scientific Meeting, 12-13 May 2016, Vancouver, British Columbia.

Barkley R, Cornila I, Atherobiotics: A probiotic designed to decelerate the progression of atherosclerosis, University of Western Ontario, Undergraduate Science Case Competition, 17-19 March 2016, London, Ontario.

Barkley, R, Koravand, A, The maturation of cortical auditory evoked potentials to verbal stimuli presented at different rates, University of Ottawa, Undergraduate Research Opportunity Project Poster Symposium, 24 March 2016, Ottawa, Ontario.

HONORS & AWARDS

2019	BioCanRX Summit for Cancer Immunotherapy Travel Grant ($1200)
2019	Canadian Institutes of Health Research (CIHR) Frederick Banting and Charles Best Canada Graduate Scholarship – Master's (CGS M) ($17500)
2019	Ontario Graduate Scholarship (OGS) ($15000)
2019	University of Ottawa Excellence Scholarship – (up to $10000)
2018	University of Ottawa Admission Scholarship – Master's ($7500)
2018	*summa cum laude* – University of Ottawa
2015 - 2018	Dean's honour list – University of Ottawa
2017	TD Green Bursaries Merit Scholarship ($1000)
2017	University of Ottawa Faculty of Science Scinapse travel grant ($250)
2017	Scinapse Undergraduate Science Case Competition third place award
2017	Scinapse Undergraduate Science Case Competition finalist ($200)
2017	Bridging Academic Minds: Science in 2025 Speaker Series second place award
2016	Scinapse Undergraduate Science Case Competition finalist ($200)
2016	Science Student Association Scinapse travel grant ($100)
2016	University of Ottawa Faculty of Science Scinapse travel grant ($250)
2015	Undergraduate Research Opportunity Program ($1000)
2013	University of Ottawa admission scholarship (annual value of $1000)

EXTRA-CURRICULAR ACTIVITIES

Intramural athletics   **September 2018 – March 2020**
University of Ottawa | Ottawa, Ontario
- Competitive ice hockey (uOttawa employee's league)

Pick-up ice hockey   **August 2018 – March 2020**
Minto Skating Club | Ottawa, Ontario

Intramural athletics   **January 2017 – May 2017**
University of Ottawa | Ottawa, Ontario
- Competitive dodgeball

Intramural athletics   **January 2016 – January 2017**
University of Ottawa | Ottawa, Ontario
- Recreational volleyball